HOT
AND
COLD
HEALTH
AND
DISEASE

ENERGETICS OF
WESTERN, CHINESE
AND AYURVEDIC MEDICINES

****

Richard G. Heft
Acupuncture Physician
Fl 1992- 2002

Disclaimer

Hot and Cold Health and Disease is based on Western, Chinese Ayurveda medicines and the questioning and counseling of thousands.

All material contained herein is provided for general information purposes only and should not be considered medical advice or consultation. **Contact a reputable healthcare practitioner if you need medical care.**

The whole is equal to and greater than the sum of its parts. **Please read the whole** book, beginning to end, and or eat the diet, first, before making conclusions about any one part.

R. G. Heft Publications
Email: rgheft@netzero.com

Hot and Cold Health and Disease (c) 2009, ISBN 0974791724 rev. 07/23/13 (paper back)

TABLE OF CONTENTS

Section IV. Daily Practices

Dedication

To the memory of my mom, and all women
The true, unsung heroes of life

Special Thanks

1. My **Mom** and **Dad** for giving me everything I needed to succeed.

2. **Dan Nevel**, Acupuncture Physician for inspiring me to study traditional Chinese medicine

3. **Dr. Richard Brown** and **Nancy Brown**, owners, teachers, Acupuncture and Massage College (formerly Acupuncture Acupressure Institute), S. Miami, FL

4. **Camillo Sanchez**, Acupuncture Physician, my first year teacher for teaching, instilling the basics

5. **Lightning Source Inc.** (printing, distributing company) the independent author's best friend

6. **Paramhansa Yogananda** (*Autobiography of a Yogi*) for bringing yoga and the wisdom of the East to the West

7. **Everyone**

INTRODUCTION
Physician heal thyself

Everyone has a dream(s). What often happens in the dream is unexpected. At age three, while sitting outside in my backyard under the sun, and putting on a band-aid, I had a vision, awakening that I was going to be a doctor despite disliking doctors (they stuck you with needles). At age ten and lasting the next 17 years was another awakening, my mother's breast cancer and subsequent medical treatment: radical mastectomy (removal of entire breast and surrounding tissue), extensive radiation, chemotherapy, pain, suffering, etc.

I often accompanied my parents on her weekend trips into the city, where I sat in the hospital, radiation ward watching my mom and others, wheeled in and out. The wheeled out was always worse, devastatingly worse. My mom suffered greatly: severe edema (elephant arms), insomnia, depression, disfigurement, etc. Her original wound, surgery, radiation burn never healed, always bled, yet the doctors were always willing to operate, medicate (chemotherapy) and radiate, whatever the risk.

At age nineteen, I took my dream to the University of Pittsburgh (1971-1974), took all the required sciences but after two years became disenchanted with the program (pre-med) as there was no discussion of diet and nutrition, which I thought was very strange. I certainly was not a medical expert but I did have common sense. I changed my major, as I felt I was wasting my time, going in the wrong direction. I took another wrong direction, major, political science (lawyer) but kept on studying health, reading diet and nutrition books.

In 1973, I read **Be Here Now** by Ram Dass (Dr. Richard Alpert). It told the story of his transformation from Western Psychologist to believer in Hinduism. I cannot say that I understood everything I read, but what I did understand were the sections on diet and yoga.

I changed my diet, from standard American (high animal protein, fat, chips, rice, pasta, bread, vegetables, fruit, soda, candy, sugar, etc.) to ovo (eggs) lacto vegetarian→ lacto (dairy) vegetarian→ vegan (no animal)→ raw foods→ fruitarian→ sproutarian (raw vegan, sprouts)→ macrobiotic (1979- 1989). The changes were immediate and positive.

For the first five years (ovo lacto to sproutarian), I felt great as I eliminated excess fat, cholesterol, water, etc. My skin became clearer. I had greater energy and was more relaxed. Then I got worse, as I lost too much weight (165 to 135 pounds), became, weak, impotent, caught colds easily, developed tonsillitis, strep throat etc. I had gone from one extreme, high protein, high fat to the other, low protein, low fat and high carbohydrate.

In 1979, I moved to Atlanta, GA and discovered the macrobiotic diet via books by Michio Kushi and a local East West Center where they taught the macrobiotic diet. I took cooking classes, learned how to cook, which was great, as prior to macrobiotics I was a lousy cook often putting foods, meals together intellectually that were nutritionally correct (vegetarian, raw, food combing, etc.) but poor in taste.

The macrobiotic diet was mostly a vegan diet (grains, beans, nuts, seeds, vegetables, land, sea, cooked, raw, fermented, etc. and fruit) with occasional fish. The food, diet really tasted good and I immediately felt better, warmer and stronger.

A year later, I moved to Brookline (suburb of Boston), MA where I attended the Kushi Institute (1980- 1981) to learn more about macrobiotics. I also got a job at Erewhon (macrobiotic wholesale company), owned by Michio Kushi. One year later, I quit and started working at the Kushi Institute.

After graduation, I moved to Langhorne, PA to manage a health food store as well as teach macrobiotics, which I did for a year before moving back to Boston, where I met my future wife. Six months later, we were married and living in North Miami Beach. FL. I got a part-time job at a local health food store Unicorn Natural Foods. A year later, I became general manager. At the same time, my wife and I taught macrobiotics (diet, philosophy, diagnosis, cooking classes, etc.) out of our home. We also had a Wednesday night dinner and lecture often attended by fifty of more people. I eventually quit my job at the Unicorn. A year later, I bought a struggling health food store in Hollywood renaming it Food and Thought.

My health unfortunately, fortunately (failure provides the seeds, motivation to succeed) got worse as I developed insomnia, eczema and a few other health problems including hair loss. Something was wrong. Whatever I was doing, eating was not right, which is why I turned to Chinese medicine and Ayurveda. Both medicines placed more emphasis on diet, herbs, exercise, etc. unlike Western allopathic medicine, which placed little or no emphasis on diet and nutrition but more on drugs, surgery and radiation.

I subsequently enrolled and later graduated the Acupressure Acupuncture Institute, Miami, FL (1989-1992) with a degree in acupuncture and related sciences, and eventually licensed professionally as an Acupuncture Physician and Nutritional Counselor (FL 1992- 2002).

I was always a diet freak, not that I wanted to lose weight, but was convinced that I could eat my way (discipline my refrigerator) to spiritual happiness, God. In my store, I always made it a point to question my customers (400+ per week) diets, always asking, "What do you eat for breakfast, lunch and dinner?" and then comparing their answers to their complaints, symptoms and diseases. My knowledge and ability to help, however was limited to macrobiotics and my own personal studies and experiences. Acupuncture school changed everything

In Acupuncture school, I learned via the theory of traditional Chinese medicine that everything, all matter is a reflection, form of **energy** that is always changing, building up (yang, hot) and breaking down (yin, cold), which in turn, changes, builds up, breaks down, thickens, thins, heats, cools, dries, moistens, expands, contracts its material form (gas, liquid, solid).

Yin and yang are the dual energetics of all matter, with one opposite, energetic temporarily in excess. There is nothing neutral, stagnant or the same. Everything is different. Differences create opposition, attraction. **Opposites attract, combine and form anew** is the creative (+) and destructive (-) force of all matter.

Atom: (elements): protons (+) and electrons (-)
Man, woman: male (+) and female (-) chromosomes
Metabolism: anabolism (+) and catabolism (-)
- Health: anabolism (building) > catabolism (cleansing)
- Disease: too much anabolism → tumors, obesity
- Disease: Catabolism > anabolism → emaciation
pH: acid (1- 7) and alkaline (7- 14) balance
- Normal, healthy blood pH, approximately 7.35- 7.45
- Disease: acidosis < 7.35, alkalosis > 7.45
Food, nutrients
- Building: hot, acidic (-), anabolic
- Cleansing: cold, alkaline (+), catabolic

Every time energy (energetic opposites) changes, its material form also changes. Controlling energetic opposites: building up (yang) and breaking down (yin) was the key to controlling, building up and breaking down, thickening and thinning, tightening and loosening, heating and cooling, stimulating and calming, drying and moistening the body, every structure function, healthy and diseased. Some opposites can be controlled, others not.

The sun and diet are the body's primary sources of energy. Every time the sun and diet change, so does the body, for better or worse.

Seasons: sun (+) and earth (-)
- Sun > earth → Spring (+), summer (++)
- Earth > sun → Fall (-), winter (--)

The **sun** (yang), day, spring and summer stimulate, heat, dry and redden the body. **Lesser sun**, night, fall and winter calm, cool, slow, contract and dry the body.

The body digests, transforms food (nutrients) and herbs into blood, structure and function. There are only two foods, nutrients: building (hot) and cleansing (cold).

I. **Building** nutrients, foods

Protein and fat (saturated and unsaturated)
(1) Red meat (highest protein, saturated fat) (2) Chicken
(3) Turkey (4) Fish (red and white) (5) Eggs
(6) Hard cheese (7) Soft dairy (8) Beans, nuts and seeds (unsaturated)

- Build, thicken, harden
- Fuel, heat, stimulate, dry redden
- Move fast, expand, rise

II. Cleansing nutrients, foods

Water, minerals, vitamins, enzymes, fiber
(1) Salt (2) Bitter herbs (includes laxatives) (3) Sugar
(4) Juices (5) Fruit (6) Vegetables (7) Grains (8) Water

- Reduce, thin, moisten
- Loosen, soften, purify
- Cool, contract, cleanse, calm, slow

Every food and herb has several tastes, major and minor. There are six tastes that adjust, heat, cool, dry, moisten, tighten and or loosen the body.

III. Six tastes

Pungent (hot, spicy) foods, herbs stimulate, heat, dry, dispels fluids (diaphoresis, sweating) and gas (carminative). Too much overheats and dries the body, blood, fluids, etc. too much.

- Onions, scallions, garlic, peppers,
- Cardamom, basil, bay leaf, cinnamon
- Ginger (fresh, dried)

Bitter foods, herbs cool, cleanse, detoxify and dry. Too much dries the body, lungs, blood, body fluids, etc. too much.

- Romaine lettuce, celery, endive
- Dandelion greens, kale
- Aloe vera, golden seal, gentian
- Barberry, turmeric, cumin, coriander

Salty foods soften dissolve, sedate, are laxative in nature. Too much weakens the kidneys, urination.

- Salt, seaweeds (high in iodine)

Sour foods, herbs heat, stimulate, nourish and dispel gas (carminative). Too much overheats, tightens the body too much.

- Lemons, limes, fermented foods, yogurt, rose hips
- Hawthorne berries, raspberries

Sweet foods heat, strengthen and dampen. Too much overheats, dampens (mucous, phlegm, cysts) the body too much.

- Animal foods, grains, fruits, sugar, ginseng

Astringent foods, herbs, cool, constrict, stop flow of blood and body fluids (sweating, diarrhea). Too much cools, contracts the body too much.

- Lemon, alfalfa, red raspberry

Food→ digestion→ **blood** → structure→ function

The body digests, transforms food, nutrients into blood. **Blood** (watery medium) carries nutrients, hormones, wastes, etc. to and from every cell, tissue via the **heart** and its vessels.

Arteries (except pulmonary) carry oxygen-enriched blood away from the heart. **Veins** (except pulmonary) carry wastes, de-oxygenated blood to the heart. **Arterioles** and **venules,** smaller branches of arteries and veins, connect to capillaries. **Capillaries** connect to all tissues, passing nutrients and receiving wastes through their thin, one-cell layer thick walls.

The quality (animal, plant, thick, thin, etc.) and quantity of food, nutrients determine the overall quality and quantity of blood, circulation, absorption and cleansing of all structure function.

All animal food (red meat, chicken, turkey, fish, eggs and dairy) contains saturated fat. **Animal protein and saturated fat** are thick, hard, sticky, damp, sweet nutrients. Too much, in the extreme, decreases circulation, causing disease.

All blood passes through the liver. The liver stores, cleanses (removes excess protein, fat, cholesterol, uric acid, etc.) and releases the blood. Too much protein, fat (especially animal) thickens the blood too much, which in turn, thickens clogs and weakens the liver. Less protein, fat, cholesterol, uric acid, etc. are removed, cleansed, more stays, thickens the blood (clots, high cholesterol), arteries, etc. The clotting factor is protein based. **Too much** protein tends to cause excess clotting.

Saturated fat contains cholesterol (essential part, nutrient of every cell, tissue, especially the brain, nerves). Too much saturated fat increases

- Blood cholesterol
- Low-density lipoproteins (LDL)
- Very low-density lipoproteins (VLDL)

LDL and VLDL harden cholesterol into **plaque**, which pastes, narrows and or blocks the arteries (atherosclerosis) reducing circulation, nutrient and waste exchange, especially in the extremities (head, arms, legs).

High animal protein, fat symptoms, diseases
- Blood clots, high cholesterol, uric acid, gout
- Poor circulation, inflammation, pain, arthritis
- Plaque, atherosclerosis, high blood pressure
- Tumors, cancer, insomnia, tinnitus (loud)
- Chest pain, angina, seizure, aneurism
- Acne, psoriasis, shingles, rashes, itching
- Dysmenorrhea, endometriosis, infertility

Too little protein, fat, in the extreme, thins the blood (blood deficiency), reduces circulation, which thins, dries, inflames, weakens and cools the body.

Low protein, low fat symptoms, diseases
- Anemia, fatigue, poor circulation
- Constipation, headaches, dizziness
- Pallor, pale lips, skin, eyelids and tongue
- Cold hands, feet, pain, inflammation, numbness
- Amenorrhea, short-term pregnancy, miscarriage
- Infertility, hot flashes, impotence, insomnia
- Autoimmune illnesses, osteoporosis, tinnitus (low)

Protein, fat and starch (processed grains, starchy vegetables) produce **nitrogen** (N_2) and **carbon dioxide** (CO_2), which are toxic, water-soluble gaseous wastes carried by the blood to the detoxifying organs. The **kidneys** filter the blood, remove N_2 in the form of urea (yellow color), and pass with urine into the urinary bladder, for eventual elimination.

Oxygen (O_2) is a vital nutrient that nourishes and purifies the entire body. The brain uses 20% of the body's oxygen content. No cell, tissue can live without it for more than a few minutes. Oxygen (water-soluble) is absorbed into the body, blood via the lungs (bronchi, alveoli).The **lungs** filter (remove CO_2) and purify (oxygenate) the blood. Long- term smoking and damp lungs (mucous, phlegm) decreases oxygen intake shortens and disturbs the breath (coughing, asthma), decreasing vitality.

The lungs are naturally moist. Water facilitates the exchange of water-soluble gases (O_2, CO_2) between the environment and the body (lungs, blood). **Too much water**, mucous, phlegm thickens, clogs and obstructs the **bronchi** (tubes) and **alveoli** (where gas exchange occurs) reducing gas exchange.

Too little water dries, weakens and narrows the lungs, bronchi, etc. Both tend to cause coughing, snoring, sleep apnea, shortness of breath, asthma and or allergies, allergic reactions to certain foods, cat hair, environmental allergens, etc

The body is naturally hot. Normal body temperature (98.6°F) **heats, dries** the body. Colder, lesser temperatures increase, thicken and slow body fluids. **Cold condenses**. In nature, colder temperatures of night and winter cool thicken moisture in the air, or on the ground into the morning dew, fog, rain (clear), snow (white flakes) or ice (clear). The body is similarly affected.

Colder body temperatures (<98.6°F) via cold, damp diet (milk, yogurt, cottage cheese, ice cream, juices, cold drinks, sugar) and environment (winter, air conditioning) **cool**, **slow** and **thicken fluids** in the lungs, throat, sinuses, breasts, vagina and uterus into

Cold, damp (wet) symptoms
- Clear or white mucous, phlegm, cysts, edema
- Copious urination, leucorrhea, yeast infection (white)
- Bacterial, viral and fungal infections (bacteria, viruses and fungi thrive in damp mediums, stagnant fluids)

Beans, cooked foods; spices, oxygen, sunshine and digestion heat the body, dry dampness. Animal foods, fish, eggs, dairy, nuts and seeds are oily, damp.

Raw fruits and vegetables (mostly water, minerals, sugar, vitamins, enzymes, fiber, require little or no digestion) cool, cleanse (dissolve, remove waste and paste) and moisten the small and large intestines, while purifying the blood. They dilute, cool and stop digestive, acid and enzyme secretion and should be eaten **last**. Eating first dilutes weakens and slows digestion.

Grains are mostly water, sugar, starch, minerals, vitamins, fiber and protein (low). They require digestive enzymes and chewing, and are less cleansing, more starch, paste (damp) when cooked, processed (noodles, bread, etc.) or not thoroughly chewed, digested. Raw, sprouted grains produce no starch, paste.

Processed or undigested grain thickens clogs, pastes and narrows the small and large intestines decreasing nutrient absorption, blood, elimination and circulation, causing painful abdominal bloating and constipation.

Every meal, diet is a combination of these basic food groups, nutrients, energetic opposites, with one energetic, nutrient always in excess. There are no neutral foods, meals, diets, symptoms, diseases, seasons, etc. **Hot, building** meals, diets in varying degrees build, thicken, energize and heat. **Less building, cold, cleansing** meals, diets, in varying degrees cool, thin, relax and drain excess protein, fat, cholesterol.

Hot, building diets +/-
- **American die**t high animal protein, fat and starch, alcohol, caffeine, low vegetables, fruit
- **Atkins** high animal protein, low carbohydrate
- **Zone** similar to middle diet
- **Ovo lacto vegetarian** dairy + eggs + vegan
- **Hot lacto vegetarian** dairy + vegan + cooked
- **Macrobiotic** vegan + seaweeds + fish

Less building, cleansing, cooling diets +/-
- **Fruitarian** fruit only
- **Sproutarian** vegan + sprouts + juices + raw
- **Raw foods** no cooked foods, only raw
- **Vegan** no animal food, byproducts, just fruit, vegetables, beans, nuts, seeds and grains
- **Cold lacto vegetarian** raw + vegan + dairy

As owner, operator of a small health food store, I regularly observed, questioned and counseled my customers (400+ per week). One question I always asked was **"What do you eat for breakfast, lunch and dinner?"** and then compared their answers to their symptoms, herbs, supplements, etc.

In the beginning, I was overwhelmed and somewhat confused by the vast number, variety of nutrients, herbs, foods, symptoms, medical diagnoses, etc. Then one day, I got it. I started thinking, seeing everything in terms of hot and cold. I noticed that those that ate drank too many hot, building foods, drinks, herbs tobacco, caffeine, tended to develop hot symptoms, diseases. Those that ate too little building or too many cold, damp foods, herbs tended to develop cold, damp symptoms, diseases.

I also realized, since there was only one body, there was only one correct diet (central theme plus two variations, and herbs) that could prevent and or cure most disease. The one diet was based on the body's nutritional composition, breakdown, ratio of building to cleansing nutrients, which was approximately **1:2, 1/3 building** 19% protein, 14% fat and **2/3 cleansing** 63% water, 4% minerals, etc.

The "middle diet" meal program is constructed accordingly, via a blend of Western, Chinese and Indian foods and herbs. Spices and herbs increase digestion and elimination of excess protein, fat, cholesterol, sugar, water, bacteria, while also heating, cooling, drying, moistening, tightening and or loosening the body. **Their use is temporary** as too much can over cool, heat, dry, moisten, tighten, loosen, build, drain, thicken and or thin the body too much causing new symptoms, diseases. There are also some herbs and spices that may conflict with prescription medications. Check with your doctor.

Middle diet, meal plan 2- 3 times per day
- **35% Protein and fat** (animal and plant)
- **15% Grain** (whole, cracked, noodles, bread)
- **50 % Vegetables** (3-5) cooked, raw and **fruit** (1)
- **Condiments**: soy sauce, Bragg's Liquid Aminos, vinegar (rice, grain or apple cider), mustard, salsa, spices, ground nuts, seeds, etc.
- **Soup** (at the beginning) and or **tea** (herb)\

The middle diet has two variations to counter the two dietary disease extremes (hot and cold). Both variations are temporary once health restores.

Variation #1 is the colder middle diet for high protein, high fat diseases, hot climates, old age and spiritual development. It is vegetarian in nature, less building, more cleansing as you cannot break down and eliminate excess protein, fat, etc., if you are still eating excess protein, fat. Expand, widen the diet (nuts, chicken, turkey, etc.) when necessary. The severity of the disease, symptoms will determine the overall strictness of the diet. Experiment as trial and error is the best teacher.

Colder middle diet, meal plan 2 times per day
- **25% Protein and fat** dairy, beans, seeds, nuts
- **15% Grain** whole, cracked
- **60% Vegetables** 3-5 per meal: 30% lightly cooked (green beans, broccoli, cauliflower, kale, collards, Brussels sprouts, etc.) and 70% raw (cabbage, celery, lettuce, cucumber, etc.) and **fruit**
- **Spices** (mild): cumin, coriander and fennel
- **Bitter herbs** aloe vera, turmeric, golden seal, gentian, barberry, burdock, dandelion, etc.
- **Beverages**: water, fruit juice, milk (dairy, non-dairy) and tea (chrysanthemum, peppermint)
- **Sweeteners:** raw sugar, maple syrup, fresh honey
- **Condiments** soy sauce (Bragg's Liquid Aminos), vinegar, mustard, ground seeds

Bitter herbs (capsules, non- alcohol tinctures or tea) are cold, contracting and drying. Suggested use: after meals, twice a day for 1- 2 weeks or more depending on results. Too much tightens, dries the body (blood, body fluids) too much causing muscle tension, pain, soreness, stiffness in chest, difficulty breathing and or nausea, vomiting, especially if taken on an empty stomach.

Variation #2 is the hotter middle diet for cold, deficient, low protein, low fat diseases and or cold climates. It is hotter, more building, heating and drying. Building foods require strong digestion. Start with smaller amounts cooked with vegetables. Gradually increase amount and frequency. Experiment and see what works, what does not. The severity of the disease, symptoms will determine the strictness of the diet.

For **cold, damp** mucous, phlegm, leukorrhea, asthma, bronchitis, edema, cellulite, Candida Albicans, yeast infections, etc. reduce and or eliminate animal foods, fish, eggs, dairy, nuts, seeds, grains (except barley, quinoa), raw vegetables and fruit. Increase beans, lightly boiled, steamed vegetables, spices, mushrooms and bitter herbs.

Hotter middle diet, meal plan 2 times per day
- **40% Protein and fat** nuts, hard cheese, eggs, chicken, turkey and or red meat
- **10% Grain** +/- Whole, cracked, noodles
- **50% Vegetables** 3-5 per meal: 70% cooked (carrots, rutabaga, hard squash, beets, parsnips, turnips), 30% raw (celery, lettuce); and **fruit** (1)
- **Spices** (basil, black pepper, cardamom, cayenne, cinnamon, cloves, garlic, ginger, etc.), **herbs** (Siberian ginseng, raspberry) and **tea** peppermint
- **Condiments** soy sauce, vegetable oil, rice vinegar, mustard and ground up seeds (pumpkin, sesame and sunflower) and nuts (walnuts, almonds, etc.)

Both diets, all food groups are adjustable. The order of eating, digestion is not. Eat from hot (soup +/- protein, fat) to cold (grain +/- vegetables + fruit). Stimulate digestion in the beginning. Cool, cleanse at the end. The middle diet will not only make you feel better but also occasionally worse as you cleanse old foods, toxins. Widen the diet to slow the cleansing process.

The following symptoms, diseases have cured by others and me via the middle diet:
- Irritable Bowel Syndrome, anal fissure, constipation
- Gastro-Intestinal Reflux Disorder, common cold, obesity
- Attention Deficit Disorder, anxiety, sinusitis, insomnia
- Plantar Fasciitis, neuralgia, miscarriage, impotence
- Acne, psoriasis, eczema, sore lower back, tooth abscess

Proper diet is the central cure for most disease, but sometimes requires assistance, in the form of nutritional supplements, herbal formulas, pharmaceutical drugs, surgery, etc. The power of remedies many times depends on the overall diet. **Example**: tomatoes and high blood pressure medications temporarily reduce but not permanently cure high blood pressure, unless you also help, by reducing animal and fried foods, while also increasing fruit, vegetables, exercise, etc.

It never hurts to see a doctor, get a medical opinion, x-rays, blood work, etc. as there are some diseases, including dietary that require medical intervention: pharmaceutical drugs, surgery, etc. The following personal story bears the painful truth and consequences (theory, practice) of well-intentioned ideas.

In my twenties, I suffered tonsillitis, strep throat every year. In 1979, I got it bad. I tried treating it with diet, herbs and acupuncture. Nothing worked. Around the 5th, 6th day, in addition to intense pain, I started hallucinating, seeing ghosts, especially during the early A.M. hours.

By the 8th day, I could barely talk or swallow. My left tonsil was completely covered with white streptococcus, swollen twice its size blocking my throat. I went, ran to the doctor. He questioned me, asked me how long this was going on. I lied, said it was only 4 days. He yelled at me, telling me how foolish I was (He was right). He told me that I was seriously ill and gave me a shot of penicillin. Twenty minutes later, when I arrived home, the swelling and strep had completely disappeared. The next day when I saw the doctor, he was amazed that I had healed so quickly, that mine was the worst case of tonsillitis he had ever seen He told me how lucky I was that I did not seriously hurt myself (burst tonsil, death).

Not seeing a doctor (penicillin) would have been a big mistake. All medicine, mainstream and alternative, has its place. Your health, life is more important than your philosophy, which may not always be right.

Over the years, I have experimented with many diets, herbs, etc. I have had many successes as well as failures. Many times, I became very sick and fortunately was able to cure. All my sicknesses turned out to be great learning experiences. Here are a few.

In 1989, I developed a bad, hideous case of eczema. It first started as a pimple, blister on my index finger (left hand) that quickly multiplied over the next few months into a multitude of blisters, cracked skin, bleeding, pus, covering every finger, the entire back of the hand and slowly moving up the back of the arm. Two fingers on my right hand were also starting to infect. I tried every Chinese herbal remedy. Nothing worked. I eventually turned to Ayurvedic Medicine. I needed to strengthen, heat my body, digestion. My diet at the time was cold, bland, sweet, low protein, low fat (soft dairy), grains, raw vegetables, tropical fruits, juices and cold drinks.

I increased animal protein, fat, cooked foods, spices and drank burdock tea, while reducing yogurt, salads, tropical and citrus fruits, juices, cold drinks, soda, etc. Within three weeks, my eczema cleared up. My digestion also got better: less bloating, gas, burping, farting, etc. I did have eczema as a teenager (not as serious).

In 2006, age 54, I developed excruciating pain in my heels. The pain was worse, especially upon rising, first thing in the morning or after sitting or lying down for any extended period, but did seem to get better with movement, exercise (walking). In the beginning, when I first started suffering, I thought I was doomed, just getting older (50's), and suffering what came naturally with age. After 7-8 months of continual pain, suffering and limping, I consulted a doctor who told me there was an operation to correct it: heel surgery to sew the loose ligaments together. This symptom, **loose ligaments** told me my condition was a circulatory disorder as my blood was **not circulating fully** to my legs, feet, ligaments, etc. (due to past high protein, fat diet, clogged arteries), which, in turn caused looseness, pain in the heels. My diagnosis was supported by the fact that my pain did get better, lesser, with movement, walking (increases circulation to the extremities: legs, arms).

I changed my diet eliminated all animal protein except turkey while increasing Swiss cheese, beans, nuts and seeds. The rest of the diet was white basmati rice, noodles, vegetables, cooked and raw (cabbage, celery), spices (fennel), fruit (apples), peppermint tea and bitter herbs (golden seal) while avoiding cooked potatoes, tomatoes (nightshades aggravate arthritis). I also ate less, spaced and or skipped meals. It took 3 months to cure, as in 100% no pain, recurrence, just long satisfying walks (2-5 miles per day) in addition to lowering my blood pressure and losing weight.

In 2013 (age 61), I changed my diet to include more cooked roots, hot spices, coffee and bitter herbs. One day, several months later I decided to have a couple of beers (hot, dry). That night I started experiencing the following symptoms: red face, increased heart rate (tachycardia), burning sensation, constriction in the chest, nausea, dizziness and fainting. A few days later my hair, became brittle, started coming out, breaking off in clumps. In two days all, the hair was gone in the back of my head. The tops and the sides also became brittle, thinned and fell out.

The cause was too many bitter herbs, coffee (bitter), hot spices, sugar and alcohol, which weakened, dried my blood, and contracted my chest producing the aforementioned symptoms. I consulted with a nurse. She checked me out, looked under my eyes, at my nails, etc. and said that I was iron deficient and that it would cause hair loss. She concluded that coffee, sugar and my long-term low protein low fat diet were contributing factors.

I immediately adjusted my diet (more milk, raw vegetables, nutritional, yeast and beans, all high in iron), stopped coffee, bitter herbs, sweets, etc. It took four days before my heart rate and blood pressure returned to normal. It would take 120 days, four months to rebuild my blood, and restore all my hair (pages 227- 8).

These case histories, mine and others, are the facts, storyline of this book that supports the theoretical basis of Chinese and Ayurvedic medicine. They work most of the time, depending on age, condition, ability to discipline, fine-tube. One thing is for sure, you never go wrong with good diet, but always go wrong with bad diet. Be flexible. Experiment; see what works, what does not.

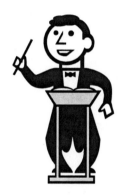

Section I. Overview

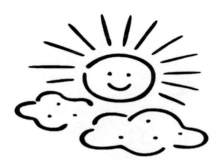

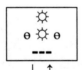

RIGHT SHOULDER	☼	**THYROID**
THYMUS RIGHT LUNG	☼	HEART LEFT LUNG
LIVER GALL BLADDER	☼	SPLEEN, **PANCREAS** STOMACH
RIGHT **ADRENAL** RIGHT KIDNEY	☼	LEFT **ADRENAL** LEFT KIDNEY
OVARIES, TESTES LARGE INTESTINE	☼	**SEX ORGANS** URINARY BLADDER

1

Chinese Medicine and Ayurveda

All matter is a reflection, form of **energy** that is always changing, building up (hot, yang) and breaking down (cold, yin), which in turn, builds up, breaks down, thickens, thins, tightens, loosens, heats, cools, expands, contracts, dries and moistens its material form. All matter is a combination, attraction and repulsion, interaction of these two energetic opposites with one opposite, energetic temporarily in excess, giving all matter its temporary energetic and material nature. There is nothing neutral, stagnant or the same. Controlling energy, building up and breaking down via diet (food, herbs), exercise, sex and rest is the key to controlling, building up, breaking down, thickening, thinning, heating, cooling, drying, moistening, the body, health and disease.

Atom: (elements): protons (+) and electrons (-)
Seasons: sun (+) and earth (-)
- Sun > earth → Spring (+), summer (++)
- Earth > sun → Fall (-), winter (--)

Man, woman: male (+) and female (-) chromosomes
Body temperature: hot (building) and cold (cleansing)
- Normal, healthy **98.6°F** (hot)
- Disease <98.6°F → coldness, shaking, autoimmune
- Disease >98.6°F → heat, fever, insomnia

Metabolism: anabolism (+) and catabolism (-)
- Health: anabolism (building) > catabolism (cleansing)
- Disease: too much anabolism → tumors, obesity
- Disease: Catabolism > anabolism → emaciation

pH: acid (-) and alkaline (+)
Food, nutrients
- Building: hot, acidic (-), anabolic
- Cleansing: cold, alkaline (+), catabolic

Opposites attract, combine and form anew is the creative and destructive force of all matter. Every time opposites attract, interact and combine, material and energetic changes occur.

The best example is the seasons produced by the earth's orbit around the sun. The **sun** (greater mass, energy) lights heats, energizes the earth. The earth (lesser mass, energy) becomes more active, productive, hot, hotter, thick, thicker, dry, drier, the closer it moves to the sun, **spring, summer** until it turns, moves away, in the opposite direction, becoming less active, cold, colder, slow, slower, thin, thinner, moist, moister, dry, drier, **fall, winter**; until it turns back, spring, summer.

The four seasons represent the **four elemental** changes, stages, transformations of all matter, produced by the interaction of yin (cold, water) and yang (hot, fire). The best example is water, which can exist as solid (ice), liquid (fluid), gas (steam) and ether (space, invisible substance). There is also a **fifth element** (earth, soil), season (late summer) that represents, symbolizes the orderly change, transition between the elements.

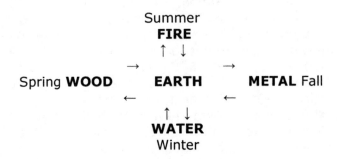

The **five elements** define the five energetic aspects of all matter: earth, body (anatomy, physiology), food, herbs, taste, emotions, colors, climates, etc.

Five Elements

	FIRE	EARTH	METAL	WATER	WOOD
Season	Summer	L. summer	Fall	Winter	Spring
Color	Red	Yellow	White	Black	Green
Climate	Heat	Dampness	Dryness	Cold	Wind
Organ	Heart	Spleen	Lungs	Kidneys	Liver
Sense	Tongue	Mouth	Nose	Ears	Eyes
Tissue	Vessels	Muscles	Skin	Bones	Sinews
Emotion	Joy	Pensiveness	Sadness	Fear	Anger
Grain	Beans	Rice	Hemp	Millet	Wheat
Taste	Bitter	Sweet	Pungent	Salty	Sour

The body, every structure function has a related, stimulating food, herb, taste, emotion, color, climate, etc. Beans, red colored foods (beets, red wine), bitter herbs and summer stimulate the heart, circulation.

Five major organs (elements) control all structure function. Energy in the body moves from one organ to another in an orderly, clockwise direction generating a **mother-son** relationship that not only nourishes (mother supports the son) but also drains (son drains the mother). Every food, herb, taste, emotion, color, season, etc. can have a positive and negative effect on the body. Know the whole before treating any one part.

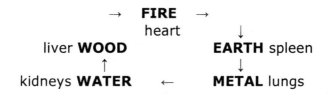

$$\begin{array}{ccc} \rightarrow \ \textbf{FIRE} \ \rightarrow & & \\ \text{heart} & \downarrow & \\ \text{liver } \textbf{WOOD} & & \textbf{EARTH} \text{ spleen} \\ \uparrow & & \downarrow \\ \text{kidneys } \textbf{WATER} \ \leftarrow & & \textbf{METAL} \text{ lungs} \end{array}$$

Fire (heart) is the **mother** of earth (spleen) and the **son** of wood (liver). Bitter foods, herbs stimulate the heart, circulation, thin, drain the blood in the heart, spleen and liver, which benefits the liver, heart and spleen when fatty, swollen, but not, when thin, deficient.

Earth (spleen) is the **mother** of metal (lungs) and the **son** of fire (heart). **Sweet foods** stimulate the spleen, pancreas, digestion and moisten the lungs, which benefit weak digestion and dry lungs not cold, damp lungs (mucous, phlegm). Too many sweet foods (sugar) weaken digestion, decrease nutrient absorption, thin the blood, weaken the heart and dampen the lungs.

There is also a **control cycle**.

- **Wood** (liver, sour) controls, **carves soil** (spleen); Too many sour foods tighten, congest the spleen, weaken digestion and bloat the abdomen.

- **Soil** (spleen, sweet) **dams water** (kidneys). Too many sweet foods dampen weaken the kidneys.

- **Water** (kidneys, salty) **extinguishes fire** (heart). Too much salt constricts the arteries, heart.

- **Fire** (heart, bitter) attacks, **melts metal** (lungs). Too much bitter dries, tightens the lungs, chest.

- **Metal** (lungs, pungent) **cuts wood** (liver). Too many spices heat, dry and tighten the liver.

The five elements are widely used in acupuncture and dietetics, but require an extensive education and years of clinical experience to fully understand, manipulate. The sun, diet and human biology are less complicated.

The **sun, spring, summer heats**, stimulates, fuels, reddens and dries the body. Lesser sun, **fall, winter cools**, calms, slows, contracts, moistens and dries.

The body digests, transforms food (nutrients) and herbs into blood, structure and function. There are only two foods, nutrients: building and cleansing.

I. Building nutrients, foods
- Protein, fat (saturated and unsaturated)
- (1) Red meat (highest protein, saturated fat)
- (2) Chicken (3) turkey (4) Fish (red and white)
- (5) Eggs (6) Hard cheese (7) Soft dairy
- (8) Beans, nuts and seeds (unsaturated fat)

- Build, thicken, fuel, heat, dry, moisten, expand

II. Cleansing nutrients, foods
- Water, minerals, fiber, enzymes, vitamins
- (1) Salt (2) Bitter herbs (3) Sugar (4) Fruit
- (5) Vegetables (6) Grains (7) Water

- Reduce, thin, cleanse, cool, moisten, dry, contract

Every food, herb also has several **tastes**, major and minor. Each taste has am overall hot or cold energetic.

- **Salty** foods (salt, seaweeds) heat, soften dissolve.

- **Bitter** foods (endive, celery), herbs (golden seal, aloe vera, gentian, turmeric) cool, dry, detox, break down fat, drain blood, fluids.

- **Pungent** foods (onions, garlic), herbs (hot spices) heat, dry and stimulate, increase protein and fat digestion, and elimination.

- **Sour** foods (yogurt, sauerkraut, lemons, limes), herbs (hawthorn berries) heat, stimulate, tighten and increase digestion.

- **Sweet** foods (grains, vegetables, fruits, sugar), herbs (ginseng) strengthen cool, dampen.

- **Astringent** foods, herbs (raspberry leaf, uva ursi) dry, constrict, stop bleeding, diarrhea, etc.

The correct balance of building and cleansing foods, nutrients, herbs, tastes maintains health. The incorrect, greater or lesser amounts, in the extreme, cause most disease via too much (thick, tight, fast, etc.) or too little (thin, loose, slow, etc.) structure function.

There are **four** dietary, disease extremes.

(1) Too much building (protein, fat) tends to cause **excess heat**: **thick, hot, yang** symptoms, diseases

- Blood clots, high cholesterol, plaque
- Atherosclerosis, high blood pressure, rashes
- Insomnia, gout, kidney and gall stones
- Fixed pain, arthritis, endometriosis, PMS
- Acne, psoriasis, warts, tumors, cancer
- Wind, shaking, trembling, paralysis

(2) Too little building tends to cause **deficient heat**, **thin, cold, dry yin** symptoms, and diseases

- Anemia, fatigue, shaking, wind (air)
- Thin, dry hair, skin, nails
- Pallor, amenorrhea, infertility, miscarriage
- Autoimmune illnesses, arthritis, dementia
- Wind, shaking, paralysis

(3) Too much cleansing, cold, damp, sweet and bitter tends to cause **excess cold**, damp, **yin** symptoms

- Abdominal bloating, gas, loose stools
- Mucous, phlegm, coughing, shortness of breath
- Asthma, cysts, edema, cellulite, diabetes
- Vaginal discharge, yeast infections, crying
- Wind, shaking, paralysis

(4) Too little cleansing tends to cause **heat, dryness**

- Dry stools, constipation, itching, scratching

Too much building and too little cleansing tend to cause excess heat, hyper-function. Too little building and too much cleansing tend to cause excess cold, damp, deficiency and hypo-function. Too little building and too little cleansing tend to cause deficiency, dryness, wind.

The treatment plan for dietary diseases is always the same. (1) Identify and eliminate the cause, extreme and (2) do the middle diet plus more of the opposite. Medical consultation, drugs, etc. may also be necessary, depending on severity.

For excess heat: colder middle diet <u>less</u> heating (salty, pungent and sour), building (spices, animal, nuts, seeds, oil), and <u>more</u> cooling (bitter, sweet), milk, beans, grains and cleansing (vegetables, fruits).

For deficient heat: hotter middle diet <u>more</u> heating (salty, pungent, sour), building (animal, nuts, seeds, oil, spices, etc.) and <u>less</u> cooling, (bitter, sweet), cleansing (soft dairy, grains, raw vegetables, fruits, juice, etc.).

For excess cold, damp modified hotter middle diet <u>less</u> bitter, sweet, animal, dairy, grains, fruits, and <u>sourer</u>, salty, pungent, beans, seeds, cooked vegetables, spices.

Yin (cold, cleansing) and yang (hot, building) and the five elements is one aspect of Chinese medicine. The **three treasures** (gunas in Ayurveda, 39- 42) are another. **Jing** (body), **chi** (mind) **and shen** (spirit) are the three essential qualities) of life.

- **Jing** is primary body substance, sexual essence (DNA, sperm, ovum), fountain of youth (strong bones, healing ability, lush hair, etc.) when full, and the onset of old age, death when low

- **Chi** is thought energy directed by the mind that transforms, transports, holds, heats and protects the body

- **Shen** is spirit (consciousness) enlivens mind

Jing (highly concentrated protein, fat) is stored in the **left kidney** (as kidney yin) and transformed by the **right kidney** (kidney yang, gate of fire) into

- Ovum, sperm, sexual organs
- Marrow, bones, brain, spinal chord
- Original chi (initial stimulus, energy of all function) floats between the kidneys

Jing is limited at birth. You only get one fuel tank, which is why conservation is important. Its decline starts soon after sexual maturity (teens to twenties) and varies according to the individual (diet, lifestyle).

Jing→ structures
- Sex organs, sperm, ovum, hormones
- Marrow, bones, brain, spinal cord
- Kidneys, teeth, head hair

Jing→ functions
- Growth, development, reproduction
- Memory, vision, hearing, locomotion
- Defecation, urination

Jing depletion: cause
- Old age, chronic illness, workaholic
- Excessive sex
- Hot, spicy foods
- Caffeine, alcohol, smoking, drugs
- Long-term anemic diet
- Extreme hot climate

Jing depletion: effect, symptoms

- Weak bones, teeth, knees, lower back pain
- Infertility, incontinence
- Dry skin, hair loss, weak vision, hearing
- Insomnia, forgetfulness, fear

Sex, masturbation, orgasm drains, *expends the greatest amount of jing*, more so in men than in women, as evidenced by the unconsciousness men tend to suffer after ejaculation, orgasm, unlike women who can experience multiple orgasms and not get tired.

Men are advised to restrain, reduce and or **forgo ejaculation**, orgasm and or sex if not pursuing children. This not only improves health, longevity but also length of lovemaking, allowing women the time needed to heat up, orgasm. The more you orgasm, the faster you age, physically and mentally. Many religions advocate celibacy and the vegetarian diet to cool reduce sexual fire, in order to grow the spiritual fire, consciousness, awareness.

Poor diet: Extreme low protein, low fat and high carbohydrate diets and impure foods **reduce** blood, **increase consumption of jing**, which is used as replacement fuel. High protein, fat diets, in the extreme, overheat, overexcite, over stimulate, over consume, burn jing. **Caffeine, amphetamines, alcohol, smoking** *and* hot climates, in the extreme, overheat dry, burn and consume jing. *Avoid hot extremes.*

Moderate lifestyle You do not want to live fast, die young. Excessive working, drinking, smoking, caffeine, sex, etc. burns jing the fastest. You do not see or feel the negative effects in the early years but instead later, in the middle years, with the early aging, graying, loss of hair, weight gain, increased ailments, etc.

Observe your grandparents. They tend to be more moderate, eat "early bird" dinners (easier to digest than late dinners). Do not wait until you are older, to act wisely eat an earlier dinner, have less sex, etc.

Deep abdominal breathing (pages 297- 300) commonly used in meditation maximizes the breath taking in more oxygen (pure chi), eliminating more CO_2, while also lowering the chi, breath, between the kidneys to unite with jing. Breathing slower, less also extends life. The more you breathe the faster you live.

Chi (energy, function) holds transforms, transports, protects and heats the body (nerves, organs, bones, blood, etc.). It is powered, built and fueled by jing, blood (nutrients, oxygen, etc.) that travel in the blood, organs, bones, nerves, meridians (energetic pathways), etc. **The mind directs chi** via thought, diet exercise, etc.

Five energetic properties of chi

- **Chi holds** the bones, muscles, organs, skin, blood, thoughts, etc. together, in their place.

- **Chi transforms** food, water, air, light, sight, into blood, bones, organs, nerves, etc.

- **Chi transports**, moves food, fluids, blood, energy, thoughts, etc.

- **Chi warms, heats** the body.

Six major types of chi within the body

- **Original chi** is the stimulus of all function

- **Primary (True chi)** is made from original and acquired chi (food, jing, blood). It transforms into nutritive and defensive (Wei) chi.

- **Nutritive ch**i is acquired chi, blood.

- **Defensive, Wei chi** is less refined and floats between the skin and the muscles. It opens and closes the pores, regulates body temperature, acts as a defensive shield in warding off environmental evils (cold, heat, wind, etc.).

- **Pectoral chi** (chest chi) nourishes the heart, lungs, throat (larynx, voice box, speech). Weak pectoral chi weakens voice, speech and respiration.

- **Organ chi** All organs have chi.

Chi is a function of fuel: oxygen, blood (protein, fat), jing (protein, fat) and space. (1) Any deficiency in fuel will cause a corresponding deficiency in chi, function. (2) Any blockage, obstruction (clots, cholesterol, tight clothing, misalignment, poor posture, injury, etc.) of space (blood vessels, bones, organs, etc.) will cause a corresponding, disruption of chi.

Four major chi pathologies mild to severe

- **Chi deficiency:** Fatigue, coldness, weak grasp, perspires and catches cold easily, shallow breathing, weak voice, chi stagnation

- **Chi stagnation**: Abdominal distention, gas, palpable lumps, pain, excess heat, higher body temperature, anger, depression

- **Chi rebellion:** Energy moving in the wrong direction: Burping, nausea, vomiting, swelling in the chest, flushing and or hot flashes

- **Sinking chi:** bruising easily, urinary incontinence, spermatorrhea (leaking sperm), varicose veins, prolapse (rectum, uterus, stomach), depression

Oxygen is a vital nutrient. It powers all function. A decrease in oxygen via lack of fresh air, polluted air, clogged lungs, sedentary life style, or poor circulation weakens decreases pectoral, lung chi. Most smokers have weak lungs, raspy voice and low vitality.

Protein and fat build and fuel all structure, function (chi). Low protein, fat diets, smoking, alcohol and caffeine decrease nutritive chi, blood, structure, function, etc.

Chi moves in defined pathways (organs, blood vessels, meridians, etc.). **Chi deficiency** slows reduces the movement of all things (food, fluids, stools, blood, etc.) as does narrowed or blocked pathways, which also tend to slow, **stagnate and or rebel** (create a backflow of energy (chi), food, fluids, burping, vomiting, etc., like a clogged and overflowing drain).

Four areas of chi stagnation:

- **Food stagnation** stomach and small intestine

- **Waste stagnation** in the large intestine

- **Blood stagnation** (clots, high cholesterol, plaque, etc.) heart, arteries, veins, etc.

- **Thought stagnation** (depression, obsession, anger, etc.)

Overeating, obesity, late night eating, Injury, tight clothing, and emotional extremes (depression, anger) tend to cause chi stagnation and rebellion (movement in the wrong, opposite direction).

Chi deficiency and stagnation are generally easy to cure via positive lifestyle changes: diet, herbs, exercise, acupuncture, massage, meditation, etc.

Long-term chi, blood, protein and fat deficiency tends to cause lack of holding **sinking chi** (prolapse, uterus, rectum, stomach, etc.). Sinking chi is chronic, more difficult to cure, requiring time, long-term dietary discipline, herbs, acupuncture and or medical treatment.

Shen is spirit consciousness, life force of the body mind. It resides largely in the brain, spine and heart. During the day, it rises into the brain stimulating thinking. At night, it sinks into the heart, where it sleeps. The ultimate goal of the shen is spiritual development, union with Spirit, God via spiritual practice: religious study, meditation, kindness, generosity, love, forgiveness, celibacy, etc. The joy, happiness of spiritual practice is greater, more lasting than the temporary joy of the body, mind and material world, which ultimately disappoint.

The three treasures (gunas) are the three mountains, tests, everyone must climb, pass. The highest mountain, test, treasure is the spirit. The lowest is the body. The mind listens to both before thinking, acting.

In Hinduism, Ayurveda, Purusha (Primal Spirit, God) is the Universal Intelligence, Consciousness that transforms into Prakruti (Great Nature, Cosmic Energy) into the

Three gunas qualities (treasures) of life

- **Sattva** spirit (shen), light, intelligence, perception, clarity, enlightenment, goodness, expansion, highest, preferred quality mind, lifestyle, etc. Meditation, kindness, fruits, vegetables increase.

- **Rajas** is mind, thought, energy (chi), activity, turbulence that can be directed up ↑ or down ↓

- **Tamas** is body (jing), darkness, obstruction, degeneration, ignorance, low quality. Animal foods, drugs, anger, greed, violence increase tamas.

Three Gunas (treasures) → 5 elements

- **Sattva** (shen, spirit) → Ether (metal)
- **Sattva and Rajas** → Air (wood, tree)
- **Rajas** (chi, mind) → Fire
- **Rajas and Tamas** → Water
- **Tamas** (jing, Body) → Earth (soil)

Five elements → 5 major organ systems (TCM)

- **Metal** → **Lungs** large intestine
- **Earth** → **Spleen, pancreas** stomach
- **Fire** → **Heart** small intestine
- **Tree** → **Liver** gall bladder
- **Water** → **Kidneys** urinary bladder

Six tastes→ organs

- **Pungent** (hot) taste stimulates, dries the **lungs**, large intestine. Too much dries, irritates.

- **Sweet** taste nourishes deficiency, stimulates **spleen, pancreas**. Too much weakens the spleen, pancreas, digestion, blood sugar, etc.

- **Bitter** taste stimulates the **heart**, moves blood, dissolve protein, fat and sugar. Too much dries, constricts the muscles, heart, blood, fluids.

- **Sour** taste stimulates the **liver**, gall bladder, and good for deficiency but not for swollen, fatty liver.

- **Salty** taste benefits **kidneys**, bladder, too much tightens; stagnates blood and overheats the body.

- **Astringent** taste regulates the colon. Too much tightens, dries the blood, fluids, constipation, etc.

The five elements produce the three doshas.

Five elements → **3 Doshas**, constitutions
- **Ether** (metal) and **air** → **Vata** moves
- **Fire** and an aspect of **water** → **Pitta** digests
- **Water** and **earth** → **Kapha** holds

Vata is air, wind that travels in the blood, arteries, veins and capillaries to the glands, organs, bones, nerves, meridians (energetic pathways), etc. Blood (watery medium) transports nutrients, chi (air, energy, vata) to every cell, tissue: Thick blood, clogged arteries and or thin (low protein, fat) blood increases wind, air, vata.

Vata symptoms, diseases (general)
- Constipation, emaciation, insomnia, dizziness
- Shaking, trembling, paralysis, debility, confusion

Increases vata
- Pungent, bitter and astringent tastes
- Dries fruits , mushrooms, fungus
- Beans, hot spices, alcohol, caffeine, smoking, sex

Decreases vata
- Sweet, sour and salty tastes, oil, dairy, animal
- Grains, nuts, seeds, cooked vegetables, fruits

Pitta is a fire, bile (digests fat). Too much protein, fat and starch (white rice, bread, noodle, cookies, chips, etc.) clog, thicken, obstruct and heat the body.

- Hunger, thirst, burning sensations, fever
- Inflammation, high cholesterol, high uric acid
- Gout, blood clots, tumors, cancer, anger
- Acne, boils, psoriasis, rashes
- Mucous, phlegm, vaginal discharge, endometriosis
- Gall and kidney stones, jaundice, insomnia

Increases pitta
- Salty, sour and pungent tastes, coffee, smoking
- Animal, fried foods, oil, alcohol, hot spices

Decreases pitta
- Sweet,, bitter, astringent tastes, bitter herbs
- Dairy, fruit, vegetables, grains, psyllium, minerals

Kapha is water, dampness (holds things together) can be hot (pitta) or cold (yin). Lower body temperatures (<98.6 F) thicken and harden body fluids into

- Mucous, phlegm, bronchitis, cysts, edema, cellulite
- Loose stools, copious urination, diabetes
- Vagina discharge, yeast infection, rashes (oily)

Increase kapha
- Sweet, salty and sour tastes, minerals
- Animal, fish, eggs, dairy, nuts, seeds
- Grains (except barley, quinoa), oil
- Fruit, juices, sodas, cold drinks, sugar, alcohol

Decrease kapha
- Pungent (hot spices) and bitter tastes
- Beans, cooked (lightly) vegetables
- Mushrooms, dandelion and chicory tea

These are all general classifications, combining Chinese and Ayurvedic medical theory. For more information: **Ayurvedic Healing** by Dr. David Frawley, O.M.D. and **Yoga of Herbs** by Dr. David Frawley, O.M.D. and Dr. Vasant Lad.

2

Energetics: biology, diet, nutrition

The body, every structure function does nothing more than build up (anabolism) and break down (catabolism) largely via diet: building and cleansing foods, nutrients and herbs. The correct balance produces health, prevents and or cures most disease via normal structure function. The incorrect, greater or lesser amounts, and poor quality foods, in the extreme, tend to cause disease via too much or too little structure function.

All matter (gas, liquid, solid) is a reflection, form of **energy** that is always changing, building up (yang, hot) and breaking down (yin, cold), which in turn, changes, thickens, thins, heats, cools, dries, moistens, expands, contracts its material form.

Building up (+) and breaking down (-) are the dual energetics of all matter with one opposite, energetic temporarily in excess, giving all matter its temporary energetic and material properties. There is nothing neutral, stagnant or the same. Differences create opposition, attraction and change. Everything at its extreme changes into its extreme. Some opposites can be controlled, others not.

- Seasons: spring, summer (+) and fall, winter (-)
- Chromosomes: male (+) and female (-)
- Food, nutrients: building (+) and cleansing (-)
- Metabolism: anabolism (+) and catabolism (-)
- pH: acid (-) and alkaline (+) balance

Opposites attract, combine and form anew is the creative and destructive force of all matter. Controlling, energetic opposites largely via diet, exercise, sexual control and rest is the key in controlling (+/-) the body, health and disease.

The **sun** and **diet** are the body's two largest sources of energy.

- The **sun, spring** (+) **summer** (++) **heats,** stimulates, fuels and dries the body.

- Lesser sun, **fall** (-), **winter** (--) **cools,** slows, contracts, moistens and dries.

The body digests, transforms food, herbs into blood, structure and function. Food and herbs contain nutrients and a variety of tastes (six) that build, fuel, heat, dry, moisten, stimulate, calm, tighten, and or loosen the body

- **Building** foods, nutrients build, thicken, fuel, heat, redden, moisten and dry.

- **Cleansing** foods, nutrients reduce, cleanse, cool and moisten.

- **Pungent** (hot) foods (onions, garlic, hot peppers, etc.), herbs, spices (cayenne, black pepper, cardamom, ginger, etc.) heat, dry and stimulate.

- **Sour** foods (lemons, limes, dairy), herbs (hawthorn berries) heat, stimulate and tighten.

- **Salty** foods (salt, seaweeds) heat, soften dissolve.

- **Sweet** foods (animal, fruits, sugar), herbs (ginseng) nourish, heat, cool and dampen.

- **Bitter** foods (lettuce, celery), herbs cool dry, detox drain fluids, dissolve fat, move down, etc.

While the sun cannot be controlled, diet (nutrients, foods, herbs) can, and is the major key to controlling, building up, breaking down, thickening, thinning, moistening, drying, heating, cooling, expanding, contracting, the body, health and disease.

Food → *digestion*→ ***blood***→ *structure*→ ***function***→

The body (stomach and small intestine) digests, breaks down food into nutrients and non-nutrients. Nutrients are transported into the blood and lymph. **Blood** (watery medium) carries nutrients, hormones, wastes, etc. to from every tissue via the blood vessels (hollow tubes) and action of the **heart** (draws and pumps blood).

- **Arteries** (except pulmonary) carry oxygen-enriched blood away from the heart.

- **Veins** (except pulmonary) carry wastes, de-oxygenated blood to the heart.

- **Arterioles** and **venules**, smaller branches of arteries, veins connect to capillaries.

- **Capillaries** connect (pass nutrients, absorb wastes) to all tissues via their thin, porous walls

The quality (animal, plant, thick, thin, etc.) and quantity of food, nutrients, and exercise determines the overall quality (thick, thin) and quantity of blood, circulation and all structure function.

I. Building protein and fat (saturated and unsaturated)

- (1) Red meat (2) Chicken, (3) Turkey (4) Fish
- (5) Eggs (6) Hard cheese
- (7) Soft dairy (milk, yogurt, soft cheese)
- (8) Beans, nuts and seeds (unsaturated)

Protein and fat (oily, greasy) build thicken and harden.

(1) Red meat (#1 blood builder, restorative for blood deficiency, in TCM) has the highest protein and saturated fat content, is more building, heating, damp and toxic (waste product) than chicken, turkey, fish and eggs. Pork is highly questionable, toxic (mucous).

(2) Chicken, **(3) turkey** and **(4) fish** (questionable, possible mercury or fecal contamination) are building, heating, oily, greasy (damp) and less toxic but easier to digest, adsorb and eliminate than red meat.

Ovo lacto vegetarian diet

(5) Eggs not considered flesh and **(6) hard cheese** are also high in protein and saturated fat, but easier to digest, eliminate. **(7) Soft cheese**: milk, yogurt, cottage cheese, ice cream contains lesser protein, saturated fat, and tend to cold, damp.

Vegan diet

(8) Beans, nuts (damp) and **seeds** (damp) are low protein; high-unsaturated fat (lowers blood cholesterol).

(9) Grains (damp, except barley, quinoa and popped grains, which drain dampness) contain small amounts of protein, little or no fat.

Protein and fat, especially animal are thick, hard, damp, sticky, sweet nutrients. Too much or too little, in the extreme, tends to cause disease.

All blood passes through the liver. The liver stores, cleanses (removes excess protein, fat, cholesterol, uric acid, toxins, etc.) and releases the blood.

Too much protein, fat, especially animal, in the extreme, tends to thicken the blood, which in turn, thickens clogs and weakens the **liver**.

Less protein, fat, cholesterol, uric acid, etc. are removed, more stays

Thickens the **blood** (clots, high cholesterol)

Blood clots (thrombus)

- The clotting factor is protein based. Too much protein tends to cause excess clotting.

Saturated fat high energy source

- Contains cholesterol (essential part, fatty of every cell, tissue, especially brain, nerves)

Too much saturated fat increases

- Blood **cholesterol**
- Low-density lipoproteins (**LDL**)
- Very low-density lipoproteins (**VLDL**)
- LDL and VLDL harden cholesterol into **plaque**

Too much plaque and clots
- Paste, narrow, clog and or block the arteries
- **Clogged, narrow arteries** (atherosclerosis) reduce circulation, nutrient and waste exchange, especially in the extremities: head, arms and legs.

Too much animal protein, fat, in the extreme,

- Thicken, inflame the **skin** (red spots, rashes, acne, warts, psoriasis, itching), **sexual organs** (tumors, dysmenorrhea, endometriosis, cancer), **brain** (insomnia, memory loss), etc.

- Clog and over stimulate the **stomach**, hydrochloric acid (HCl): nausea, heartburn

- Clog, overheat, dry and foul the **large intestine**: dry stools, constipation, foul odor, tumors, cancer

Too little protein and fat thins the blood. **Thin, low protein, low fat blood**, in the extreme, tends to

- Reduce circulation, cold hands and feet

- Dry, thin or crack the **skin, hair, nails, bones**

- Easily bruise, bleed

- Cause **arthritis**, pain, inflammation, weakness, numbness, shaking in the joints, muscles, etc.

- Cause **autoimmune illness**, eczema, insomnia, memory loss

- Cause amenorrhea, **infertility**, miscarriage, short-term pregnancy, impotence, fear, depression

Animal protein, fat quickly rebuilds, corrects blood and chi (energy) deficiency. It is best served with vegetables, herbs and spices to counteract its hot, thick, sticky, acidic, toxic (waste) nature. Animal food especially flesh (1- 3) is difficult to digest, eliminate, especially when consumed with starch. **Cloves, spices and bitter herbs** help digest and detoxify animal flesh.

Milk, yogurt and soft cheese contain less protein, fat and tend to be cold, damp, mucous forming especially when served with additional cold, damp foods (grains, especially processed, fruit, juices cold drinks, sugar, etc.).

Cottage and Swiss cheese create lesser mucous. **Goat milk** is easier to digest than cow milk (difficult to digest, best drunk alone, primarily food for cows, babies, not adults). Yogurt digests well with fruit. Soft dairy eaten with sugar, starch (cereal) tends to cause abdominal bloating, gas and sour body odor. Ice cream is a dietary nightmare (cold, sugary and fatty). **Spices** (cardamom, cinnamon, ginger, etc.) help digest dairy.

One animal protein per meal is easier to digest, eliminate than two or more. Whatever you do not digest, eliminate, you store (obesity, cholesterol, tumors, etc.). Animal flesh benefits those (1) living in cold climates, (2) doing hard physical labor or (3) suffers blood deficiency.

Eat quality foods. Free range, organically fed, hormone, antibiotic, pesticide and preservative free animals are healthier and less toxic than commercial. **Read labels**

Nuts, seeds are best ground and eaten raw (easier to digest). Do not cook. **Beans** are difficult to digest, unless soaked overnight, sprouted, served raw or cooked with *spices and sea salt, at end when soft.* All are high in **unsaturated fatty acids** and high-density lipoproteins **(HDL)** that help dissolve and eliminate excess protein, fat, cholesterol, etc. Too much unsaturated fat lowers HDL. Seeds, nuts and beans (nourishing, moistening) benefit the bones, hair, skin, nails, etc.

The sun, protein, fat, cooked foods, spices and digestion fuel, heat the body, increasing body temperature. Normal body temperature ($98.6°F$) heats, regulates (thins) bodily fluids (mucous, urine, etc.). Colder body temperatures via long-term cold, damp diet or climate **cool, thicken**.

Cold condenses. In nature, colder temperatures condense, thicken and harden water in the air or on the ground into the morning dew, rain (clear), snow (white flakes) and or ice. The body is no different.

Lower, colder body temperatures less than 98.6°F via cold, damp diet (soft dairy, fruit, cold drinks, etc.) and climate **thicken and harden** fluids in the lungs, throat sinuses, breasts, vagina and uterus into

- Clear or white (snow) mucous, phlegm
- Coughing, snoring, hacking
- Shortness of breath, asthma, sleep apnea
- Sour body odor, breath
- Cysts, edema
- Vaginal discharge, yeast infection
- Glossy facial (ice cream) complexion

II. Cleansing water, minerals, vitamins, enzymes

- (1) Salt, minerals (2) Bitter herbs (laxatives)
- (3) Sugar (4) Fruit (5) Vegetables
- (6) Grains (7) Water

- Cool, moisten, soften, loosen, calm
- Reduce, cleanse, sink, contract, move slow

Grains contain very little protein, fat and are primarily water, minerals, sugar, etc. Processed (noodles, bread, etc.) and cooked grains are dry, starchy, sticky, pasty. Too much (includes cooked, starchy vegetables) tends to **paste, clog and harden** the intestines:

- Hard, painful, abdominal bloating, gas
- Pasty stools, rashes
- Appetite (via decreased nutrient absorption)
- Weight gain, higher body temperature, etc

Whole grains, soaked, sprouted and eaten raw are easier to digest and eliminate. Many cultures crack, mill their grains, remove the outer husk, before cooking, making them more digestible, as does chewing (mixes grain with saliva, ptyalin digestive enzyme for starch).

Raw vegetables and fruits are mostly water, minerals, sugar, fiber, vitamins and enzymes. Fruit contains more sugar Cooking decreases water while increasing starch in vegetables. *Fiber* like a broom sweeps away paste, waste in the small and large intestines.

All waste products (undigested food) are toxic (poisonous), and require daily elimination to prevent re-absorption back into the bloodstream. Vegetables contain more fiber and are therefore more cleansing. There are three kinds of vegetables. A balanced meal should have all three, minimum 3- 5 (cooked and raw).

1. **Above ground, leafy greens**: kale, collards, watercress, carrot tops, etc. soothe the lungs.

2. **Ground level**: cabbage, broccoli, cauliflower, celery, onions, summer squash, etc. lightly cooked or raw soothe, cleanse the middle, round organs (stomach, spleen, liver, gall bladder).

3. **Below ground, roots**: carrots, daikon radish, burdock, beets, parsnips, turnips, rutabaga, etc. and roots soothe the intestines, kidneys, bladder and sex organs. Too many (cooked) can overheat the body.

Raw vegetables and fruits are cold, damp; require little or no digestion (acid, enzymes). They cool, stop digestion, secretion of acid, enzymes, cleanse the intestines, and generally eaten at the end of the meal.

Too many, especially at the beginning weakens, dilutes and slows digestion (abdominal bloating, gas) and elimination (loose stools) while reducing nutrient absorption, blood.

Cooked vegetables (more starch, less water), soups and stews are more warming, stimulating, grounding and appropriate (easy to digest) for those with cold, weak digestion or live in a cold, damp climate. Cooked foods heat the body. Raw vegetables, fruits, juices and cold drinks cool, dampen the body, and generally eaten at the end of the meal, day. They also make better nighttime snacks than bread, cookies, chips, etc.

Fruits and vegetables are sweet, sugary. Regular consumption helps reduce sugar cravings, especially concentrated sweets (cookies, pastries) and sweeteners.

Concentrated sweets and sweeteners (honey, molasses, sugar, fructose, maple syrup, etc.) are cold, damp, absorb quickly, instantly increasing (temporarily) blood sugar, and energy. Unfortunately, the energy, blast of concentrated sweets, sugar is short-lived unlike protein, fat, which is stronger, longer.

Overeating especially protein, fat, starch and sugar overworks, weakens the pancreas: hyperglycemia, hypoglycemia, diabetes, hyper, and or hypo activity. The pancreas (produces digestive enzymes and insulin) regulates digestion and blood sugar. Proper diet and herbs restore the pancreas, depending on severity.

The best quality food (plant, animal) is organically grown, no pesticides, herbicides, preservatives, colorings, hormones, unlike commercial (non-organic) produce from large farms, which is generally highly contaminated.

Eat organically grown when possible Washing, light cooking, boiling helps kill and eliminate bacteria and other water-soluble pesticides, herbicides, etc. in commercial produce. Discard the cooking water. Buy in 3-5# packages, which significantly reduce the cost. Taste and nutrition are more important than variety.

Every meal, diet is a combination of building and cleansing foods, nutrients, with one opposite nutrient, always in excess. There are no neutral meals, diets, etc. The following tables list common diets accordingly.

Hot, building diets +/-
- American diet high animal protein, fat, starch, alcohol, caffeine, sugar, low vegetables, fruit
- Atkins high animal protein, low carbohydrate
- Zone similar to middle diet
- Ovo lacto vegetarian dairy + eggs + vegan
- Hot lacto vegetarian dairy + vegan + cooking
- Macrobiotic vegan + seaweeds + fish

Cleansing, cooling diets +/-
- Fruitarian fruit only
- Sproutarian vegan + sprouts + juices + raw
- Raw foods uncooked, fermented
- Vegan no animal food, byproducts, just fruit, vegetables, grains, beans, nuts, seeds, etc.
- Cold lacto vegetarian dairy + vegan + raw

The correct diet, balance of building and cleansing is determined by the body's nutritional composition, ratio of building to cleansing nutrients, which is approximately **1:2, 1/3 building** and **2/3 cleansing**. The middle diet, meal plan is constructed accordingly. Asian and many American restaurants regularly serve this diet, in one form or another. The following are general guidelines.

Middle diet, meal plan 2- 3 times per day
- **35% Protein and fat** (animal and plant)
- **15% Grain** (whole, cracked, noodles, bread)
- **50% Vegetables** (3-5) cooked, raw, and **fruit**
- **Soup** (in the beginning) and or **tea** (at the end)
- **Condiments** +/- spices soy sauce, vinegar, etc.

The middle diet, meal plan has two variations to balance, treat the two dietary disease extremes. The two variations including spices and herbs are temporary until health restores, at which time the middle diet resumes. The number of meals one eats depends on one's condition. High protein, fat diseases may only require two meals per day, and low protein, fat diseases, three.

The colder middle diet helps counter, balance high protein, high fat diseases, hot climates and old age. Small amounts of chicken and turkey are permissible, especially in the colder months, fall and winter. Decrease dairy, nuts, grains, oil, fruit and juices if damp, kapha (page 42)

Colder middle diet, meal plan 2 times per day
- **25% Protein and fat** dairy, beans, seeds, nuts
- **15% Grain** whole, cracked
- **60% Vegetables** 3-5 per meal: 30% lightly cooked (green beans, broccoli, cauliflower, kale, collards, Brussels sprouts, etc.) and 70% raw (cabbage, celery, lettuce, cucumber, etc.) and **fruit** (apples, pears, pineapples, figs, dates)
- **Spices** (mild): cumin, coriander and fennel
- **Bitter herbs** aloe vera, turmeric, golden seal, gentian, barberry, burdock, dandelion
- **Beverages**: water, fruit juice, milk (dairy and non-dairy) and tea (chrysanthemum, peppermint)
- **Sweeteners:** raw sugar, maple syrup, fresh honey
- **Condiments** soy sauce (Bragg's Liquid Aminos), vinegar, ground seeds

Colder middle diet, sample meals
- Soy cheese, bread, lettuce, celery, apple, tea
- Walnuts, noodles, cooked broccoli, cauliflower, raw celery and lettuce, soy sauce, fruit
- Rice, mung beans, carrots, celery, broccoli, parsley, cumin, coriander and fennel, fruit
- Millet, cooked buttercup squash, onions and potatoes, ground sesame seeds, soy sauce
- Barley, adzuki beans, cauliflower, raw potatoes, celery, walnuts, raisins, fennel, cumin, coriander, turmeric, soy sauce (Bragg's), etc.
- Vegetable noodle soup: lightly cooked broccoli, cauliflower, raw celery, parsley, fennel, cumin, coriander and ground walnuts. Cook noodles separately (follow directions on package).

Add spices Organic, non-irradiated) at the end of cooking, as they require no digestion. Bitter herbs (capsules, tinctures (alcohol and non-alcohol) and bulk in tea form) are generally consumed at the end, or after a meal, not on an empty stomach as their cold, contracting nature may cause nausea and or vomiting. If so, drink hot water. Bitter herbs, except turmeric decrease intestinal flora. Turmeric combines well with other bitters.

Bitter herbs (includes green tea) are contraindicated for deficiency, vata conditions. Too much weakens, dries the blood, tightens the chest, etc. **The standard recommendation** is 1- 2 times per day for 1- 2 weeks or more as long as you are getting positive, healthy results. Discontinue when getting negative, unhealthy responses: headaches, constipation, abdominal pain, insomnia, chest pain, muscle tightness. Alcohol tinctures aggravate excess heat, yang, pitta and vata conditions. Put in hot, boiled water for a few minutes, which will dissipate, eliminate the alcohol.

Most herbs except relaxants (sleeping, calming) are taken during the daytime. More information: **Ayurvedic Healing** by Dr. David Frawley, O.M.D., **Yoga of Herbs** by Dr. David Frawley, O.M.D. and Dr. Vasant Lad **and Energetics of Western Herbs, Volumes I, II** by Peter Holmes. Medical consultation may be necessary as *some herbs may conflict with prescription medications.*

The hotter middle diet, for breakfast and lunch benefits, helps counter cold, deficient, damp diseases and those living in cold climates. Spices increase digestion, warmth, energy treat the common cold, stomachache, diarrhea, worms and parasites. Suggested use is three to seven per meal with food. Eat a light dinner (vegetarian). For **cold, damp** mucous, phlegm, leukorrhea, asthma, bronchitis, edema, cellulite, Candida Albicans, yeast infections, etc. reduce and or eliminate animal foods, fish, eggs, dairy, nuts, seeds, grains, raw fruit, juices (all damp), while increasing beans, vegetables (lightly boiled, steamed), hot spices, mushrooms, bitter herbs. The severity of the disease, symptoms will determine the strictness of the diet. Experiment and see which foods, herbs makes you better or worse.

Hotter middle diet, meal plan 2 times per day
- **40% Protein and fat** nuts, hard cheese, eggs, chicken, turkey and or red meat
- **10% Grain** +/- whole, cracked grains. Decrease bread, cookies, chips
- **50% Vegetables** 3-5 per meal: 70% cooked (carrots, rutabaga, hard squash, beets, parsnips, turnips), 30% raw (celery, lettuce); and **fruit** (1)
- **Spices, hot** (basil, black pepper, cardamom, cayenne, cinnamon, cloves, garlic, ginger, etc.), **herbs** (Siberian ginseng, raspberry), **tea**
- **Condiments** soy sauce, vegetable oil, rice vinegar, mustard and or ground up seeds, nuts

Hotter middle diet, sample meals
- Chicken, walnuts, rice, mixed vegetables, fruit
- Turkey, onions, turnips, carrots, raw lettuce, celery, turmeric, cumin, coriander. fruit, green tea
- Vegetable omelet, black pepper, turmeric, toast, jelly, fruit, green tea
- Cheese sandwich, cooked, raw vegetables, fruit

Hot spices benefit cold, damp (kapha) condition, but in excess tend to cause dryness, itching, insomnia, etc. Mild spices (fennel, cumin and coriander) and bitter herbs benefit hot (pitta) conditions. Too many spices dry the body, blood too much itching, inflammation, irritation, anemia, insomnia, etc. Anything can be done to excess, extreme. Extremes cause disease. Use what works improves your health. Discontinue what worsens.

The primary food groups, spices, herbs, etc. can always be adjusted, increased or decreased according to one's needs (condition, climate, etc.). **When in doubt, eat simply**: protein, vegetables and fruit.

Drinking with meals should be kept to a minimum (soup, water and or tea). Cold drinks, sodas, ice tea, fruit juices, etc. dilute and weaken digestion (acid, enzymes) and elimination, especially when drunk at the beginning of the meal. Drink when you are thirsty. If not thirsty, do not drink. Eight glasses of water per day generally benefits the overheated, working outdoors or live in a hot climate, not the cold, damp or live in a cold climate. The best quality water is running, filtered (removes impurities including fluoride).

Eat from hot (soup, protein and fat) to cold (vegetables and fruit) to increase digestion, nutrient absorption and elimination. Eating fruits and vegetables first, decrease digestion, nutrient absorption.

The stomach should be approximately **½ solid, ¼ liquid and ¼ empty** to allow the moving and mixing of food and fluids. One plate of food per meal is advised. **Overeating** clogs, slows the movement of food, decreases digestion, absorption and elimination. As one gets older, eat less: two meals per day, snacks. Periodic fasting on fruit juice, one day per week is generally beneficial as it allows non-food sources of energy to heal and energize the body.

Avoid rigidity. Everything (age, condition, climate, etc.) changes. Today's diet, herbs, exercise, etc. may balance today's age, condition, climate, etc. but not necessarily tomorrow's age, condition, climate, etc. Be flexible in diet, exercise thought, etc.   Consult with a doctor. Do what you feel is right.

The middle diet while balanced is extreme, in contrast to the way most people eat. It may cause rapid healing, discharging of accumulated poisons into the bloodstream, sickening the body, cleansing organs, etc. too fast, which is why the diet may need widening (old foods, junk, etc.) to slow the healing process.

Diet is very powerful in the treatment of most disease but many times requires additional help, supplementation: nutritional, herbal, pharmaceutical drugs, surgery, etc. depending on severity. Too much supplementation weakens. All medicine has its advantages and disadvantages. **Ultimately, the *patient decides* treatment**. It is everyone's right.

The only person who can cure you is you. The smarter, more intelligent (read books) and disciplined you become the greater your chances of maintaining health, curing disease. Drugs, alcohol, caffeine, overeating, etc. weaken will power.

3

Vitamins, Minerals and Enzymes

Vitamins, minerals and enzymes play an important role in the assimilation of nutrients and all bodily functions. Most can be derived from food and herbs. The best quality foods, organically grown without the use of synthetic fertilizers, pesticides, herbicides, artificial food colorings, antibiotic and hormone free are preferable, as they provide the best quality, vitality, nutrition. Nutritional supplements (natural better than synthetic) taken with food can also be beneficial. For more information, please read **Prescription for Nutritional Healing** by Phyllis Balch, CNC and James Balch, M.D.

Vitamins, which represent less than one percent of our body make up, are essential for normal growth, development and metabolism. They have a broad range of functions: building up (anabolism) and break downing (catabolism) all body tissues, releasing nutrients and stored energy from digested food, etc.

There are two types of vitamins: **water-soluble** (B complex and C) which must be taken daily as they are not stored and **fat soluble** (A, D, E and K) which need not be taken daily, as they are stored in the body and live for longer periods of time. Water-soluble vitamins are heat sensitive and generally destroyed by cooking.

Vitamin A (includes carotenoids) benefit the eyes, skin, immune system, bones and teeth. A deficiency of Vitamin A can manifest as night blindness, dry hair and skin, fatigue, insomnia and skin disorders.

Carotenoids (carotenes) are a precursor to vitamin A. The liver converts them into Vitamin A. Both forms of Vitamin A have high antioxidant properties, which protect the body from harmful free radicals, cancer, etc. Free radicals damage the cells reduce immunity and cause infections and various degenerative diseases.

Too much Vitamin A, more than 100,000 international units (IU) per day can damage the liver, spleen, hair, reproductive organs, skin, etc.

Food and herbal sources of Vitamin A
- Fish liver oils, animal livers
- Dark leafy greens (kale, collards, dandelion, beet)
- Carrots, spinach, yellow squash, sweet potatoes
- Spirulina, kelp, peaches, apricots
- Alfalfa, burdock, cayenne pepper, horsetail, sage

B Complex benefits the eyes, skin, hair, nerves, brain, liver, mouth and energy production. There are ten different B Complex vitamins that work together, which is why they should generally be taken together, although they can be taken individually for short periods. A deficiency of one B vitamin in general indicates a deficiency of the entire B complex.

Vitamin B_1 (thiamine) benefits the brain, circulation, blood formation, production of hydrochloric acid (digestion), carbohydrate metabolism, and counters the effects of alcohol and smoking. A deficiency of B_1 tends to cause beriberi (nervous system disorder), constipation, fatigue, edema, difficulty breathing, nervousness and or numbness.

Food and herbal sources of Vitamin B_1
- Egg yolks, fish, poultry, brewers yeast, kelp
- Dried beans, nuts, brown rice, raisins
- Alfalfa, burdock, nettle, peppermint, raspberry

Vitamin B2 (Riboflavin) aids in the formation of red blood cells, antibody production, carbohydrate, protein and fat metabolism, cell respiration, helps eliminate dandruff, prevent cataracts and benefits pregnancy. A deficiency of B2 tends to cause eye disorders, inflammation, cracks and sores at the corners of the mouth, dermatitis, dizziness, insomnia, and or hair loss.

Food and herbal sources of Vitamin B2
- Meat, chicken, egg yolks, fish, cheese, milk
- Broccoli, leafy green vegetables, mushrooms, kelp
- Alfalfa, burdock, horsetail, peppermint, raspberry

Vitamin B3 (Niacin, Nicotinic acid, Niacinamide) benefits the nervous stem, skin, circulation, digestion (production of hydrochloric acid and bile), carbohydrate, protein and fat metabolism, and helps lower cholesterol. A deficiency of B3 tends to cause diarrhea, indigestion, loss of appetite, low blood sugar, muscular weakness, fatigue, dizziness, insomnia, pellagra and or canker sores. Niacin tends to cause flushing of the skin. Avoid taking if pregnant, diabetic, suffering glaucoma, high blood pressure and gout. Check with your doctor before using.

Food and herbal sources of Vitamin B3
- Fish, eggs, cheese, brewers yeast
- Broccoli, carrots, tomatoes, wheat germ, kelp
- Alfalfa, burdock, horsetail, peppermint, raspberry

Vitamin B5 (Pantothenic Acid) aids in the production of neurotransmitters, adrenal hormone, antibodies; helps convert protein, fat and carbohydrates into energy, and is the known as the "anti stress" vitamin. A deficiency of B5 tends to cause headaches, fatigue, nausea and or tingling in the hands.

Food sources of Vitamin B5
- Beef, eggs, brewers yeast, nuts, fresh vegetables

Vitamin B6 (Pyridoxine) aids in the production of red blood cells, hydrochloric acid (HCl), absorption of Vitamin B12, protein and fat, helps maintain sodium potassium balance and normal brain function. A deficiency of B6 tends to cause headaches, nausea, vomiting, anemia, inflammation of the gums, acne, arthritis, dizziness and or fatigue.

Food and herbal sources of Vitamin B6
- Meat, chicken, fish, eggs, brewers yeast, kelp
- Beans, brown rice, walnuts, peas, spinach

Vitamin B12 (Cyanocobalamine) aids in the metabolism of carbohydrates and fat, production of red blood cells, helps prevent anemia via absorption and utilization of protein, folic acid and iron. It also helps fertility, maintains myelin nerve sheaths, prevents nerve damage and improves sleep. A deficiency of B12 tends to cause malabsorption, digestive disorders, constipation, pernicious anemia, bone loss, chronic fatigue, depression, dizziness, palpitations and or ringing in the ears. Deficiency symptoms may not appear right away, as Vitamin B12 is stored in the body for up to five years. Some vegetarians tend to suffer from B12 deficiency.

Food sources of Vitamin B12
- Fish, eggs, dairy, brewers yeast
- Sea vegetables, soybeans

Biotin aids carbohydrate, protein and fat metabolism, utilization of B vitamins, sleeping and benefits the nerves, bone marrow, hair and skin. A deficiency of biotin tends to cause anemia, high blood sugar, muscle pain, depression, hair loss and or insomnia.

Food sources of biotin
- Meat, poultry, egg yolks, milk, brewers yeast
- Whole grains, soybeans

Choline benefits the nerves and brain (transmission of nerve impulses and the protective sheaths surrounding the brain and nerves), hormone production, liver (reduces fat) and gall bladder function, lecithin (lipid) formation (major substance of cell membranes that regulate passage of nutrients), helps digest cholesterol and prevent arteriosclerosis and cardiovascular disease. A deficiency of choline tends to cause gastric ulcers, inability to digest fats, fatty buildup in the liver and or high blood pressure.

Food sources of choline
- Meat, egg yolks, soybeans, lecithin, whole grains

Folate (folic acid) aids in the formation of red blood cells, fetal development (pregnancy), brain, immunity (increases white blood cells), protein, metabolism, energy production and cell division, replication. A deficiency of folate tends to cause anemia, fatigue, birth defects, gray hair, insomnia, forgetfulness, and sore red tongue.

Food sources of folate
- Beef, chicken, tuna, cheese, milk, brewers yeast
- Whole grains, beans, dark leafy green vegetables
- Root vegetables, mushrooms, wheat germ

Inositol aids in the formation of lecithin, metabolism of fat, helps reduce cholesterol, hardening of the arteries (arteriosclerosis); and is vital for hair growth. A deficiency of inositol tends to cause high cholesterol, arteriosclerosis and or hair loss.

Food sources of inositol
- Meat, milk, brewers yeast, lecithin
- Whole grains, beans, vegetables, raisins

Para-Aminobenzoic Acid (PABA) helps maintain intestinal flora, assimilate B5 and protect against sunburn.

A deficiency of PABA tends to cause fatigue, indigestion, nervousness, and white patches of skin and or graying of the hair.

Food sources of PABA
• Liver, kidney, whole grains, spinach, mushrooms

Vitamin C (Ascorbic Acid) is an antioxidant that benefits adrenal gland function, anti-stress hormones, immunity (counters pollution, free radicals and toxins in the blood, protects against infection, fights cancer), reduces low-density lipids (bad cholesterol) and heavy metals, increases high-density lipids (good cholesterol), lowers high blood pressure, helps prevent arteriosclerosis, abnormal blood clotting and bruising. A deficiency of Vitamin C tends to cause indigestion, fatigue, bleeding gums, tendency to easy bruise, low resistance to infections, common cold, scurvy; poor wound healing and or tooth loss. Vitamin C (acidic) is best taken in its buffered form (with minerals).

Food and herbal sources of Vitamin C
• Citrus fruits, green vegetables, kelp
• Alfalfa, fennel, horsetail, peppermint, raspberry

Vitamin D is fat-soluble that acts both as a vitamin and hormone that benefits the immune system and the proper functioning of the thyroid. It is also necessary for the absorption and utilization of calcium and phosphorous, important in the growth and development of the bones and teeth, especially in children.

There are several forms of Vitamin D. D_2 is found in food. D_3 is synthesized by the skin, which reacts to the sun's ultraviolet radiation. It is the most common form of Vitamin D. Exposure to the sun twenty minutes per day is more than sufficient. Severe deficiency can cause rickets in children, insomnia, osteoporosis, visual problems, etc.

Food and herbal sources of Vitamin D
- Fish liver oils, fish, eggs, milk, butter, oatmeal
- Vegetable oils, nettles, horsetail, parsley

Vitamin E is an antioxidant that improves circulation, blood clotting, healing, reduces blood pressure, increases sperm production, promotes healthy nerves, skin and hair, helps prevent anemia, cardiovascular disease and cancer, and retards aging, oxidation via the inhibition of free radicals. A deficiency of Vitamin E tends to weaken red blood cells, cause infertility, menstrual problems, miscarriage, and or nerve deterioration.

Food and herbal sources of Vitamin E
- Eggs, milk, beans, nuts, seeds, whole grains
- Cold pressed vegetable oils, dark leafy greens, kelp
- Alfalfa, dandelion, raspberry leaf, rose hips

Vitamin K is essential in the production of prothrombin, which aids blood clotting. It also helps bone formation, repair and converts glucose to glycogen, storage form of sugar in the liver, which aids liver function. A deficiency of Vitamin K tends to cause abnormal bleeding (internal and external).

Food and herbal sources of Vitamin K
- Egg yolks, yogurt, blackstrap molasses, oatmeal
- Dark, green leafy vegetables, kelp
- Alfalfa, green tea, nettles

Vitamin P (Bioflavonoids) helps absorb Vitamin C, promote circulation, protects the capillaries, relieves pain, bruises, stimulates bile production, lowers cholesterol and helps treat cataracts.

Food sources of Vitamin P
- Peppers, black currants, grapes, plums, prunes
- White skin beneath peels of citrus fruits

Minerals make up 4% of our body's total weight and are vital in the formation of blood, nerves, bones, muscles, body fluids, etc. It is best to get them from food rather than supplements; however, supplements also have their advantages. Take with food, especially in the evening, as they have a calming, sedative effect. Taken on an empty stomach may cause nausea. *Some minerals may conflict with prescription drugs*. Check with your doctor. Caffeine and sugar tend to deplete minerals.

Boron in trace amounts helps build the brain, bones (helps prevent postmenopausal bone loss), muscles and aids in the metabolism of calcium, magnesium and phosphorous. A deficiency of boron tends to cause Vitamin D deficiency.

Food sources of boron
- Nuts, whole grains, leafy greens, carrots, apples

Calcium helps build strong bones, teeth, strengthens the nerves, heart (maintain heartbeat, lowers cholesterol, blood pressure), gums, muscles, blood (aids clotting), digestion (increase enzyme activity) and may prevent cancer. A deficiency of calcium tends to cause muscle cramps, numbness in the arms and legs, joint pain, rickets, tooth decay, brittle nails, high cholesterol, high blood sugar, palpitations and or insomnia. Coffee and sugar deplete calcium weaken the bones, teeth, nerves.

Food and herbal sources of calcium
- Fish, dairy, brewers yeast, kelp, almonds
- Dark leafy green vegetables, sesame seeds
- Alfalfa, chamomile, fennel, flax, horsetail, nettle

Chromium aids in the metabolism of glucose (sugary form of energy) helps maintain blood sugar levels, as well as synthesizing of protein, fat and cholesterol.

A deficiency of chromium, also known as the glucose tolerance factor (GTF) tends to cause fatigue, anxiety and blood sugar problems. Chromium picolinate is the best, most absorbable form, supplement. *Do not use if you are insulin dependent.* Check with your doctor.

Food and herbal sources of chromium
- Meat, chicken, eggs, cheese, brewers yeast, dulse
- Whole grains, beans, blackstrap molasses
- Horsetail, licorice, nettles, oat straw, wild yam

Copper aids in the formation of hemoglobin, red blood cells, nerves, bones, joints, skin (coloring) and hair. A deficiency of copper tends to cause anemia, baldness, osteoporosis, diarrhea and skin sores. Take with other minerals as too much copper may adversely affect the eyes, vision.

Food sources of copper
- Fish, nuts, beans, barley, broccoli, leafy greens
- Mushrooms, radishes, blackstrap molasses, oats

Germanium is a carrier of oxygen, helps oxygenate the cells, eliminate toxins, poisons, while improving immunity.

Food and herbal sources of germanium
- Milk, shitake mushrooms, broccoli, celery, onions
- Aloe vera, ginseng

Iodine (in trace amounts) benefits the thyroid gland, helps prevent goiter and aids in the metabolism of fat. A deficiency of iodine tends to cause mental retardation in children, fatigue, hypothyroidism and weight gain. Too much may inhibit the secretion of thyroxin (thyroid hormone) producing swollen salivary glands, diarrhea, vomiting and **metallic taste** or sores in the mouth.

Food sources of iodine
- Fish, dairy, kelp, iodized sea salt, sesame seeds
- Soybeans, lima beans, spinach, garlic, asparagus

Iron aids in the production of hemoglobin and the oxygenation of red blood cells. It is the largest mineral found in the blood. It also aids energy production and the immune system. Inadequate dietary intake, poor digestion, menstruation, blood loss, long-term illness, excessive coffee and tea, too many bitter herbs, sugar, and a diet high in phosphorous (page 69) tends to cause iron deficiency. Do not take iron supplements if you are not anemic. A deficiency of iron tends to cause anemia, pallor, fatigue, nervousness, dizziness, brittle hair, hair loss, fragile bones, deformed nails (spoon shaped, horizontal ridges) and or indigestion.

Food and herbal sources of iron
- Meat, poultry, fish, eggs, brewers yeast, kelp
- Whole grains, green leafy vegetables, almonds
- Lima and kidney beans, sesame seeds, pumpkins
- Peaches, pears, raisins
- Alfalfa, dong quai, fennel, horsetail, licorice, nettle

Magnesium aids enzyme activity, energy production, helps prevent soft tissue calcification, maintains pH balance, strengthens the muscles and used as a stool softener. A deficiency of magnesium tends to cause poor digestion, insomnia, rapid heartbeat, hypertension, seizures, heart disease, irritability and or diabetes.

Food and herbal sources of magnesium
- Meat, fish, dairy, eggs, brewers yeast, kelp
- Whole grains, soybeans, green leafy vegetables
- Apples, apricots, grapefruit, peaches
- Alfalfa, cayenne, horsetail, licorice, nettle, parsley

Manganese (trace amounts) benefits the nerves, bones, cartilage, synovial fluid (lubricate the joints), reproduction, mother's milk, immune system helps regulate blood sugar, benefits iron deficiency anemia and aids in the metabolism of protein and fat, A deficiency of manganese (rare) tends to cause vision and hearing problems, high cholesterol, atherosclerosis, hypertension, raid pulse, memory loss and or tremors.

Food and herbal sources of manganese
- Egg yolks, whole grains, nuts, seeds, beans
- Seaweed, green leafy vegetables, pineapple
- Alfalfa, dandelion, chamomile, horsetail, parsley

Phosphorous benefits the blood (clotting), bones, teeth, heart, kidneys, and helps covert food into energy. Excessive intake interferes with calcium absorption. Take with magnesium and calcium. A deficiency of phosphorous (found in many foods) is rare.

Food sources of phosphorous
- Poultry, eggs, fish, dairy, brewers yeast
- Whole grains, nuts, seeds, beans, dried fruit
- Seaweed, green leafy vegetables, pineapple

Potassium benefits the blood, nutrient absorption, nervous system and heart (maintains heartbeat, blood pressure, helps prevent stroke), and works with sodium to maintain water balance. A deficiency of potassium tends to cause diarrhea, constipation, dry skin, acne, edema, thirst, insomnia, high cholesterol, low blood pressure, muscular fatigue and or salt retention. Tobacco and caffeine reduce potassium absorption.

Food sources of potassium
- Meat, poultry, fish, dairy, brewers yeast
- Whole grains, vegetables, fruit

Selenium is a powerful antioxidant especially when combined with Vitamin E. It benefits the heart, liver, pancreas and immune system, inhibits the oxidation of fats (lipids) and the formation of free radicals. Free radicals damage age the body. It also regulates thyroxin, thyroid hormone (regulates fat metabolism) and helps prevent the formation of tumors, especially affecting the lungs, colon and prostate. A deficiency of selenium tends to cause infections, liver and pancreas dysfunction, exhaustion, growth impairment and or high cholesterol. Too much selenium tends to cause hair loss, brittle nails, metallic taste, garlicky breath, pallor, tooth loss and or arthritis.

Food and herbal sources of selenium
- Meat, chicken, dairy, brewers yeast, kelp
- Whole grains, vegetables, Brazil nuts
- Alfalfa, fennel, horsetail, nettle, parsley

Silicon aids in the production of collagen (protein of connective tissues) which benefits the bones, cartilage, nails, skin and hair, aids calcium absorption, counters the affects of aluminum, softens the arteries, increases immunity and slows the aging process.

Food and herbal sources of silicon
- Whole grains, soybeans, leafy greens, beets
- Alfalfa, horsetail and silica supplements

Sodium benefits the stomach, nerves and muscles helps maintain water balance and blood pH (acid alkaline balance). Sodium deficiency is rare although can be brought upon low sodium diets and excessive use of diuretics. A deficiency of sodium tends to cause anorexia, dehydration, abdominal cramps, headache, dizziness and heart palpitations. Too much tends to cause edema, potassium deficiency and high blood pressure.

Sulfur cleanses, disinfects the blood (chemicals, pollutants), protects, kills harmful bacteria, counters radiation, benefits the skin and slows the aging process.

Food and herbal sources of sulfur
- Fish, eggs, beans, wheat germ
- Cabbage, onions, turnips, kale
- Horsetail and MSM (supplement)

Zinc benefits the prostate, reproductive organs, immune system, bones, skin, taste and sense of smell. A deficiency of zinc tends to cause the loss of smell and taste, fingernail deformation (thin, cracked, white spots), hair loss, acne, delayed sexual maturation, infertility, impotence, prostate disease and weak immunity, healing

Food and herbal sources of zinc
- Meat, poultry, fish, egg yolks, brewers yeast, kelp
- Beans, whole grains, pumpkin and sunflower seeds
- Alfalfa, burdock, chamomile, dandelion, fennel

Enzymes (energized protein molecules) benefit all biochemical activities within the body. There are two types of enzymes: digestive and metabolic.

Digestive enzymes break food down into its smallest component parts: nutrients and non-nutrients. Nutrients are absorbed directly into the bloodstream via villi and lacteals in the small intestine. They are secreted in the mouth, stomach and small intestine.

There are three main classes of digestive enzymes: amylase, protease and lipase. **Amylase** in saliva, pancreatic and intestinal juices breaks down carbohydrates. **Protease** in the stomach, pancreatic and intestinal juices breaks down protein. **Lipase** in the stomach and pancreatic juices breaks down fat.

Metabolic enzymes govern chemical reactions within the cells, especially energy production and detoxification. They help construct nutrients into the body, individual tissues. The two most important are super oxide dismutase (SOD) and its partner catalase. SOD is an antioxidant that attacks free radicals. Catalase breaks down hydrogen peroxide (metabolic waste) while releasing oxygen.

There are tens of thousands of enzymes within the body. However, twelve major enzymes control the digestion and assimilation of carbohydrates, protein and fat.

Enzymes are also heat sensitive. Cooking destroys all enzymes, which is why a raw foods (fruits, vegetables, etc.) are a necessary part of the diet. Supplementation may also be necessary, as enzyme production decreases with age.

Food sources
- Apples, bananas, mangos, papayas, pineapple
- Avocados, sprouts (very high)

Papayas and pineapples contain proteolytic enzymes: papain and bromelain. Alfalfa, wheat and barley grass, sprouts and cabbage are high in SOD.

4

Spices and Food Grade Chinese Herbs

Spices and food grade Chinese herbs aid regulate digestion, elimination, fluids and energy. Digestion, digestive fire (acid, enzymes) cooks, breaks food down into nutrients and non-nutrients.

- Nutrients → bloodstream → structure function
- Whatever food, fluids not digested absorbed becomes waste→ large intestine, urinary bladder

Weak digestion via long-term low protein, low fat diets or too many fruits, juices, cold drinks, overeating, in addition to tight clothing, sitting or lying down after meals decreases digestion, nutrient absorption, slows the downward movement of food in the stomach, small intestine (bloating, gas, heartburn and nausea) and large intestine (loose stools, constipation).

Chronically weak digestion or deficient blood cools the body. Colder, lower body temperatures (<98.6°F) cool and harden bodily fluids into mucous, phlegm, edema, cellulite, cysts, discharges, yeast infection, and or sour, sweet or musty body odor.

Most spices are heating; stimulate digestion, move energy, heat the body, dry dampness, anti-bacterial, destroy and eliminate poisons, etc. The use of spices varies according the individual (condition, climate, etc.).

Spices

- **Increase digestion**, burning of excess protein, fat, cholesterol, thins the blood

- **Increase perspiration**, which cools the body, relieves common cold, sore throat, muscle tension.

- **Best served with food**, especially fruit, vegetables (sweet), grains, beans, desserts, soups, stews, etc. Ground spices require no cooking.

- **Caution, contraindication**: Spices may worsen, overheat and dry existing hot, dry conditions: itching, scratching, sore throat, dry cough, etc.

There are several categories, energetic classifications of spices. For more information please read **Ayurvedic Healing** and **Yoga of Herbs** by Dr. David Frawley O.M.D., **Energetics of Western Herbs Vol. I, II** by Peter Holmes and **Spices** by John Heinerman

1. Carminatives increase digestion, are spicy, bitter, drying, reduce excess fluids (mucous, phlegm, cysts, edema, cellulite, loose stools, etc.) while dispersing food stagnation (abdominal bloating, gas, heartburn, nausea). Stagnant fluids are a common growth medium for many bacteria, viruses and fungi.

- Garlic, coriander, cumin and chives

2. Stimulants increase circulation of blood and energy, disperse excess fluids, food stagnation in the intestines.

- Black pepper, cayenne pepper, cinnamon bark
- Cloves, fresh (less hot) and dried ginger
- Fennel (less hot)

3. Aromatic herbs, spices are warm, spicy, fragrant, dry dampness (mucous, phlegm, loose stools); stimulate the pancreas (digestive enzymes). The aromatic smell in the blood, body odor is offensive, toxic and repelling to many bacteria viruses and mosquitoes. All spices are aromatic.

4. Spicy, warm and bitter herbs release the surface

- Oregano, basil and ginger are spicy, warm herbs that cause diaphoresis (perspiration).

- Peppermint and spearmint are spicy bitter (cold), treat shoulder, neck tension sore throat (mild), colds (onset) and toothache (peppermint oil).

5. Asafetida and turmeric aid in the digestion of beans. Turmeric (bitter taste) stimulates the liver and gall bladder, increasing the flow of bile (emulsifies, digests fat, especially eggs).

Chinese food grade herbs

Build, move or drain (1) chi (energy, function), (2) blood, and (3) fluids. The following is a general list of Chinese food grade cooking herbs (includes Chinese Mandarin name), most of which are edible. **Inedible herbs will be marked with an asterisk (*).**

Many Asian groceries (Chinese, Vietnamese) **carry these herbs**. *Please consult with a physician before using* any of these herbs. You do not have to eat the herbs, just cook, strain (into a separate cup) and drink the broth. Start with small amounts.

(1) Dried tangerine peels *(Chen pi)* drain damp moves phlegm reduces bloating and gas.

---

(2) Astragalus (Huang qi)* stimulates the spleen, digestion, drains excess water (mucous, phlegm) and strengthens the immune system, fights colds. It is contraindicated when excess heat, infection.

(3) Lotus seeds (Lian zi) build energy; nourish spleen, kidneys, treat incontinence of sperm, urine, vaginal secretions, etc. Soak 6- 7 seeds overnight or ground into powder and cook. In the whole form, the cooking time (presoaked) is 30 minutes+ until soft.

(4) Red dates (Hong zao) nourish energy, blood, fluids and the spleen (digestion). They are contraindicated when there is phlegm in the lungs. They also have pits (remove prior to cooking). Cook dates (5) 10 minutes.

(5) Dioscorea (Shan yao), wild yam strengthens the spleen, stomach (digestion), kidneys and lungs, treats coughing (dry, no mucous), bed-wetting, diarrhea, diabetes, poor appetite, weak digestion, especially infants. Ground dioscorea into powder (1-3 pieces), added to food, and cooked for 10 minutes.

(6) Lily bulb (Bai he) moistens the lungs, dry cough while moving phlegm. Presoak a small amount (TB) for ½ hour and then cook 15 minutes.

(7) American ginseng (Ren shen) increases blood, energy, immunity, libido, digestion, moistens the lungs, more appropriate for the elderly (dryness) as it is not as heating or drying as other ginsengs. General use is 2-3 pieces in tea or food (30 minutes +/-).

(8) White peony (Bai shao yao) * balances the liver, regulates menstruation, reduces irritability, tinnitus dizziness. Cook 3-5 pieces 10 min.

(9) Korean and Chinese ginseng (Panax) grow on opposite sides of the mountains separating Korea and China. Energy tonics (more warming), strengthens lungs and immune system while quieting the mind.

(10) Black dates (Da zao) nourish the spleen, stomach strengthen energy, blood, while calming the mind. Contraindicated when phlegm in the lungs. Black dates have pits. Cooking time 10 minutes (5 pieces).

(11) Poria (Fu ling) is a fungus that helps eliminate excess damp (mucous, phlegm, edema, diarrhea), generally contraindicated for yeast or fungal infection. Cook (small amount) 10- 15 minutes

(12) Lycii berries (Gou qi zi) nourish blood, essence, eyes, vision and treats indigestion, diarrhea, anemia and nervousness.

(13) Fresh ginger (Sheng jiang) is hot, sweet and moistening. It increases digestion, circulation and helps eliminate cold, damp, mucous, phlegm, coughing and gas. Cook several slices 5+ minutes or grate 1TB in tea, food. Dried ginger is hotter, drier, may be too drying for chronic deficiency conditions.

(14) Rhemannia, cooked (Shu di huang) nourishes blood, kidneys, regulates menstruation, treats anemia, dizziness, palpitations, insomnia and is contraindicated when there is dampness. Cook small amount 10-15 min.

(15) *Codonopsis (Dang shen)* is similar in effect to ginseng, known as poor man's ginseng. It increases energy, fluids, and strengthens the spleen, stomach, bones and muscles. General use is 3- 4 pieces. Cook 15- 20 minutes.

(16) Longan fruit (Long yan rue) nourishes blood, essence, invigorates the heart, spleen, and treats insomnia, dizziness, palpitations and forgetfulness. Cook 5-10 minutes

(17) Angelica sinesis (Dang gui) builds, circulates blood, and regulates menstruation. Cook small amount 10 minutes, contraindicated during pregnancy.

(18) Fo ti (He shou wu) nourishes blood, kidney and liver essence and helps restore hair color. Cook 15 minutes alone (tea), or with other foods, especially black beans.

(19) Black fungus (Hei mu erh) nourishes blood and essence, moistens the intestines (good for constipation) and helps to lower cholesterol. Contraindicated: dampness, yeast

(20) Black mushrooms (Xiang gu) drain damp, clean, moisten the intestines (dry constipation) and aid the immune system and contraindicated when there is dampness, yeast. Cook 30 min. +/- according to size.

5

Cooking Class

While there are many good cooks, restaurants, the best cook, restaurant, is you in your own kitchen. If you can buy, wash and cut vegetables, boil water, add spices, follow a recipe and keep track of time you are ready to be a cook. You will need a minimum of 10- 30 minutes +/- per meal. Welcome to the world's shortest cooking class, based on the middle diet.

Middle diet, meal plan
- **35% Protein and fat** (animal and plant)
- **15% Grain** (whole, cracked, noodles, bread)
- **50% Vegetables** (3-5, cooked, raw) & **fruit** (1)
- **Soup** (beginning), **tea** (end)
- **Condiments:** ground nuts and seeds soy sauce (Bragg's), vinegar (rice, grain, apple cider), mustard, salsa, spices and round nuts, seeds

You can find this menu in any Asian (steamed with the sauce on the side) and many American restaurants (be creative). The middle diet, meal plan is the traditional way of eating that mimics the body's natural, nutritional composition, ratio 1:2

- **1/3 building**
- **2/3 cleansing**

Digestion and absorption are also important, as all food, nutrients not digested, absorbed become toxic waste. Poor diet, sedentary lifestyle reduces digestion, absorption and elimination.

The hardest foods, nutrients to digest are protein and fat, especially animal, which requires stronger and longer digestion in the stomach and small intestine. The stomach produces hydrochloric acid (HCl) and other enzymes specifically designed to digest animal protein, fat. Pancreatic enzymes and *bile* from the pancreas and *liver* via pancreatic and *gall bladder* ducts (tubular connections) digest food in the small intestine.

The sun, protein, fat, cooked foods and spices stimulate digestion, production of acid, enzymes. Raw vegetables, fruits (mostly water, minerals, sugar, etc., require little or no digestion, processing) cool, stop digestion while cleansing, eliminating waste, are generally eaten last.

Order of eating
(1) Soup +/- protein and fat
(2) Protein and fat +/- grain
(3) Grain and vegetables (cooked then raw)
(4) Fruit and tea (end)

Eat from hot (building) to cold (cleansing)

The stomach (7- 9A.M.) and small intestine (1- 3 P.M.) are highly charged, strongest during the day, early morning and afternoon, and weakest after the sun goes down. Eat protein, fat at the beginning of the day, meal to take advantage of the sun, stomach and small intestine, and vegetables, fruit and tea last. Stimulate in the beginning, cool, cleanse at the end. Eating cold, sweet foods: sugar, fruit, raw vegetables first dilutes, weakens digestion, absorption, blood, elimination, etc.

Eat more during the day, less at night

Nutrient absorption into the bloodstream and lymph takes place in the small intestine (22 feet)

Eating early meals and being upright (gravity) several hours after eating improves the downward movement, spreading of food increasing digestion, nutrient absorption and elimination. Eating late decreases digestion absorption, elimination, while increasing waste. If you eat it at night, you will most likely wear it in the morning, in the intestines, arteries, skin, waist, thighs, etc. Eat more vegetables, fruit in the evening to, cool, calm, than protein and fat, which heat, stimulate (insomnia).

Cooked versus raw foods

Digestion is a fiery process that cooks, transforms, food, nutrients into blood, while also destroying harmful bacteria, parasites, etc. Cooking aids the digestive process. A certain amount of cooking is beneficial, grounding for most people, as is a certain amount of raw, depending on one's condition, climate, etc. Cooking decreases water, increases starch (paste) in vegetables.

High quality foods

Organically grown (no chemical pesticides, fertilizers, dyes, waxes, preservatives, hormones, antibiotics, etc.) fruits, vegetables, grains, beans, nuts, seeds, free range, antibiotic and hormone free dairy, poultry and red meat are the best quality (more nutritious) and tastiest. Most commercial produce, meats, etc. are generally tainted (colorings, preservatives, antibiotics, hormones, etc.)

You never go wrong sicken with high quality foods. You can buy organically grown foods at most neighborhood supermarkets and or health food stores. The price drops significantly when you buy bulk (3- 5#). Organic farming is environmentally, earth friendly as it replenishes the soil with "natural foods" old produce, grass cuttings, manure, etc.

Fresh food is more nutritious than canned, preserved, frozen or day old food. You can also buy or filter your own water if you do not trust municipal water, fluoridation. Poor quality food produces poor quality health, disease.

Cooking pots and utensils are important. Use cast iron, stainless steel, enamelware and glass pots in addition to wooden cooking utensils (do not scratch, less noisy). Certain materials (Teflon, aluminum, etc) tend to scratch, chip easily and can leach hazardous chemicals into your food. Do not buy Three Mile Island potteries. Cooking pots with thicker bottoms evenly distribute the heat, unlike thin bottoms, which do not.

Cooking classes and cookbooks are also essential, informative and social. Learn how to cut, layer vegetables, make soups, stews, desserts, etc. Check the local newspapers and health food stores, for cooking classes. There are also many good cookbooks on the market. I like Mary Estelle's **Natural Foods Cooking**. The best teacher is your own experience: trial and error.

Every meal will have the same basic structure (middle diet):
- **1/3 protein, fat** animal, plant
- **1/6 grain** optional
- **1/2 vegetables, fruit**

Cooking times vary. Meat, chicken, eggs, etc. take 5-60 minutes to cook. Leftover, cooked chicken, turkey etc. takes less time. Beans and whole grains, in general, can be soaked overnight to decrease cooking time or sprouted and eaten raw. Cracked grains and noodles (follow directions) take less time. Some meals may take as little as 10 minutes, others 30 minutes+.

Vegetables cut into smaller pieces (matchsticks, slivers, diced, etc.) tend to cook faster than larger sizes. You can layer the vegetables, onions first on the bottom, then roots (carrots, burdock, turnips, etc.), then ground and aboveground (leafy greens). The vegetables on the bottom receive more heat; cook faster than the top, which cook slower. Avoid frying.

Soups are easy to make. Add grains, beans, vegetables, etc. to a pot of water, cover and bring to a boil for the required time. Grains and beans take a longer time to cook than vegetables. Add vegetables towards the end. Root and ground vegetables have a longer cooking time than aboveground, leafy greens vegetables. Light vegetables (celery, cabbage, etc.) can be cooked for one minute or less or added raw (more nutritious) add a crunchy texture. Add spices and other condiments (soy sauce, oil, rice vinegar, etc.) last or place on the table, as they require little or no cooking. Soups are easy to digest.

I. SOUPS

Lentil soup (28 minutes)

1. Add ¾ C washed lentils to 4- 6 C water
2. Cover; bring to a boil, reduce flame, simmer, **cook 20 minutes+** until beans soft.
3. Add ½ onions, 1 carrot. **Cook 5 minutes**
4. Add a few pinches of sea salt (after beans are soft). Salt (minerals) increases fat digestion. Adding salt at the beginning prevents them from swelling, cooking, softening. **Cook 2 minutes.**
5. Add 2 celery stalks, spices: cumin, coriander and fennel. Mix, **turn off flame**.
6. Add ground walnuts, 1 tsp. sesame oil, soy sauce (Braggs Liquid Aminos) and rice vinegar. Garnish with parsley. **Serve**

This is a basic bean soup recipe. You can add, subtract, and change any ingredient. Be sure to adjust cooking time. Adzuki, black, kidney, chickpeas, navy, and turtle beans generally take one hour+ to cook. You can soak these beans overnight to decrease cooking time or sprout and add at the end (step 6). Rice vinegar aids in the digestion of beans, and combined with sesame oil produces a creamy flavor, taste.

2. Cabbage, corn, celery, onion soup (6 min)

1. Add onions and corn to 4- 6 C of water. Cover and bring to a boil. **Cook 5 minutes.**
2. Add celery, cabbage. **Cook 1 minute**
3. **Turn off flame.** Add spices (cumin, fennel, etc.), walnuts, 1TB sesame oil, soy sauce and or rice vinegar. Garnish with parsley. Serve

3. Vegetable and grain soup (27 minutes)

1. Add ¼ C white basmati rice, 1/8 C fresh corn, few pinches of sea salt to 4- 6 C water
2. Cover; bring to a boil and then simmer (lower the temperature, flame), **cook 20 min+**, until soft.
3. Add onions and carrots. Cut thin, small (cooks faster). **Cook 3 minutes.**
4. Add broccoli, cauliflower. **Cook 2 minutes.**
5. **Turn off flame**. Add spices: cumin, coriander, fennel, turmeric, cayenne, etc. ground pecans, 1tsp sesame oil, soy sauce (Braggs Liquid Aminos) and rice vinegar or the condiment of your choice. Garnish with parsley, scallions. Serve.

You can substitute or mix any grain. Cooking time is always the longest grain. Brown rice, barley, whole oats, etc. take 45 minutes+ to cook. Millet takes 20 minutes. Cook until soft. Salt aids digestion of grain.

The following are general breakfast menus, suggestions. Each food group is adjustable according to one's taste, condition, climate, etc.

II. Breakfast menus

1. Oatmeal, raisins and walnuts (8 minutes)

1. Mix ¼-C oatmeal flakes (rolled) to ¾-C water. Cover, lower the flame, ***cook 7-9 minutes***. Cooking longer with extra water softens grains
2. Add walnuts, raisins with a few pinches of cinnamon at the end of cooking.

Soft cereals are generally easy to digest. You can add raisins, ground walnuts, sunflower seeds, spices, red dates (have pits), sea salt (pinch), soy sauce, etc. You can also use leftover grain to make a soft cereal, porridge, congee (longer cooking). Sea salt is the best quality salt (more trace minerals).

2. Vegetable omelet (10 minutes)

1. Oil the pan with vegetable oil or butter. Turn on the flame. Add 3- 5 vegetables (broccoli, carrots, celery, cauliflower, etc.) with 2-3 eggs. **Cook 5- 8 minutes**, or go out to a restaurant. Eat someone else's food. Finish with green tea.

3. White rice, hard-boiled eggs, broccoli, onions and carrots (25 minutes)

1. Add 1/8 cup of rice and pinch sea salt
2. Add 1½- 2 cups of water, cover, bring to a quick boil and lower flame, **cook 20 minutes**
3. Add onions, carrots, broccoli and two raw eggs (in the shell). **Cook 5 minutes**

4. Take eggs out of the pot and remove the shells. Add eggs back to the pot.
5. Add spices (black pepper, turmeric)
6. Finish with green tea helps digest fat

4. Chicken or turkey, vegetables and white basmati rice (30 minutes)

1. Add 1/8 C of rice, pinch of sea salt to 1½- 2 C of water, cover and *cook, simmer* **20 minutes+**
2. Add broccoli, carrots, precooked chicken, turkey or meat. **Cook 3- 5 min.**
3. Add raw celery, cabbage, potato (sliced thin), and spices: black pepper, turmeric, fennel, etc. and or condiments. Mix and serve.

5. Swiss cheese (sliced) raw romaine lettuce, celery and potatoes (with skin) and fruit (apple, orange, etc.) simple but quick meal that gives you flexibility in protein (beans, nuts, eggs, chicken, and turkey), vegetables (cooked, raw) and fruit.

The following lunch and dinner menus are mostly vegetarian. If you need more protein, fat, substitute turkey, chicken or cheese. You can also substitute grains, beans, seeds, nuts, vegetables, fruits, etc.

III. Lunch and Dinner menus

1. Millet and tempeh stew (25 minutes)

Cooking pot #1
1. Add ¼ cup of millet, pinch of sea salt to 2 cups of water (+/-). Cover, bring to a boil, then lower flame, simmer and **cook 25 minutes**. Mix with #2

Cooking pot #2

1. Add sliced onions, carrots, black mushrooms (presoaked 1/2 hour) and 3 ounces of tempeh to 4 cups of water. Cover, **cook, simmer 15 minutes**.
2. Add celery, zucchini (cubed), potatoes (minced), walnuts, spices and soy sauce. Serve with pot #2
3. **Mix** with millet (pot #1)

2. Adzuki beans, barley and vegetables (62)

Cooking pot #1

1. Add 1/8 cup each adzuki beans, barley, 5 lotus seeds (soak overnight) to 4 cups of water. Cover, **cook, simmer 1 hour** *until soft*
2. Add sea salt and raisins. **Cook 2 minutes**
3. Add spices, 1TB soy sauce and serve with pot #2

Cooking pot #2

1. Add broccoli, carrots, cauliflower to 2 C of water (+/-), cover, lower flame, **cook 3- 5 minutes**
2. Add raw celery (1-2 stalks, sliced), cabbage and pecans. **Cook 1 minute**. Serve with pot #1

3. Noodles, black beans and vegetables (60)

Cooking pot #1

1. *Add* 1/8 cup black beans (soak overnight, discard liquid), 1 strip kombu seaweed to 3 C of water+. Cover, lower flame and **cook 45 min.**
2. Add onions and squash (buttercup). **Cook 20 min.**
3. Add sea salt. **Cook 3 minutes**
4. Add raw celery, cabbage, spices cumin, turmeric and coriander. **Cook 1 minute** Serve with pot#2
5. Add precooked noodles (follow directions, **boil 4- 10 minutes** until done.
6. Add ground sesame or sunflower seeds, soy sauce and rice vinegar

You can also substitute rice, add ground walnuts, pecans, etc. change vegetables, condiments, etc. You do not have to eat grain (whole, cracked, noodles, bread) with every meal. Skipping grain is a great way to lose weight.

4. Mung beans, walnuts and vegetables (33)

Cooking pot #1
1. Add 1/8 cup: mung beans to 2C water. Cover, bring to boil then lower flame, **simmer 30 min.**

Cooking pot #2
1. Cook, s*auté on*ions, **2-3 minutes**
2. Add cabbage, celery. **Cook 1 minute**
3. Add walnuts, spices, rice vinegar, soy sauce
4. Combine with pot#1 and serve

5. Tofu, noodles and vegetables (10 min)

Cooking pot #1
1. Add ¼ brick tofu (cut into cubes), onions, and parsnips (cut thin) to 2 C of water (+/-). Cover, bring to boil, lower flame. **Cook 5- 8 minutes**
2. Add raw celery, ground walnuts, fennel, cumin, coriander, 1TB soy sauce, etc. Serve with pot #2

Cooking pot #2
1. *Boil* noodles in 2C water, for **3- 10 minutes** (follow directions).Strain excess water, rinse with cold water and mix with pot #1

Desserts (simple fruit to cookies, cakes, pies, etc.) are sweet and served at the end of the meal. Complex desserts are not a feature of every meal. If they are then they will also be a feature of every waistline.

V. Desserts

1. **Cous cous cake** (serves 2) Combine ½ C each: cous cous and apple juice with raisins, walnuts and a little cinnamon. Bring to a boil; turn off the flame, cover, wait 10- 15 minutes, serve.

2. **Agar agar** (seaweed gelatin) Boil 1 tsp. agar flakes (comes with directions) in ½ to 1 cup apple juice. Add nuts and dried fruit. Bring to a boil and stir until the agar flakes have disappeared. Turn off the flame, cover and put into the refrigerator. Let sit ½ hour.

3. **Fruit compote** Cook bananas, apples, pears, walnuts and raisins together 5 minutes. Season with spices, cinnamon, cloves, etc. Great way to use up left over and or bruised fruit.

4. **Cookies** Buy any cookie mix and add a pre cooked baked yam (without the skin), grated carrots or apples into the mix. This not only increases the size of the batch but also sweet taste (reduces need for concentrated sweets). My good friend Marcia came up with the idea.

These are natural desserts. Sometimes they are not sweet enough which is why there is junk food. Sometimes, you need a little junk to help counter the junk, stress of life. Normally the best dessert is fruit. If you eat too much dessert, and or overeat, eat Kim chi (Korean pickled spicy cabbage), raw cabbage (fiber, enzymes), carrots and or apples (fiber, pectin, enzymes) at the end, to digest, move and eliminate sweet, sticky, doughy, oily, greasy food. Hot tea increases protein and fat digestion.

V. Herbal teas

1. **Green tea** (bitter, contains a slight trace of caffeine) aids fat digestion and helps lower cholesterol. It may cause nauseas on an empty stomach. Do not flavor with sugar, sweeteners.

2. **Chrysanthemum** aids in the digestion of fat (oil) and benefits the liver, heart, arteries and prostate

3. **Hawthorne berry** aids digestion, helps lower cholesterol and blood pressure.

4. **Bancha twig** helps digest protein and fat.

5. **Peppermint and spearmint** tea aid digestion, help remedy sore throats, loose stools and toothache. Do not boil mint teas. Add hot water to tea, let sit for a minute, then strain.

The kitchen is your digestive system. Digestion transforms and transports food, nutrients into blood. Keep the kitchen clean and active. A healthy kitchen produces a healthier bedroom. An unhealthy kitchen dooms the bedroom.

Variety is not a necessity. You do not have to eat every fruit, vegetable, grain, cheese, chicken, turkey, etc. You can have a repertoire of ten vegetables, five fruits, three or four beans, seeds, nuts; one kind of cheese, turkey, etc. Balance, not variety is the key.

Cooking while healthy can often get tiring which is why eating at restaurants on occasion is necessary just as it is occasionally necessary to eat junk food. The healthier you eat, feel the lesser your tolerance, desire for junk food, overeating, etc.

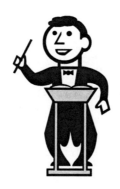

Section II. Biology

Everything is a product of cause and effect. You reap what you sow

Cause→ effect
Input→ output

Hot, dry diets, climates → hot, dry symptoms
Hot, damp diets, climates → hot, damp symptoms
Cold, dry diets, climates → cold, dry symptoms
Cold, damp diets, climates → cold, damp symptoms

6

Blood and Body Fluids

Food→ Digestion→ **Blood**→ Structure→ **Function**→

The body builds up and breaks down (cleanses) largely according to food, nutrients. Nutrients are transported, absorbed into the bloodstream, lymph. **Blood** carries nutrients, hormones, wastes etc. to and from every cell, tissue, structure function via the **heart** and its vessels (arteries, veins and capillaries). The body also transforms nutrients and non-nutrients into **body fluids** (mucous, urine, synovial, etc.) which moisten, lubricate.

Five major organ systems regulate blood, body fluids and all structure function.

Spleen-stomach
- Digestion, blood

Heart-small intestine
- Blood, circulation, digestion

Liver-gall bladder
- Digestion, blood cleansing

Lungs-large intestine
- Respiration, blood cleansing, elimination

Kidneys-urinary bladder
- Reproduction, blood cleansing, elimination

The **heart** commands (pumps, moves) the blood and its vessels (tubes). **Arteries** (except pulmonary) carry oxygen-enriched blood away from the heart. **Veins** (except pulmonary) carry de-oxygenated blood to the heart. Smaller branches of arteries and veins **arterioles** and **venules** connect to capillaries.

Capillaries connect to the tissues, passing nutrients and receiving, absorbing wastes through their thin, porous one-cell layer thick walls.

The quality and quantity of food, nutrients and non-nutrients determines the overall quality and quantity of blood, circulation and all structure function.

Animal protein and fat (saturated) are thick, hard, sticky nutrients that build, thicken, fuel, heat. Too much or too little, in the extreme, tends to cause disease (hot and cold)

All blood passes through the liver. The liver

- **Cleanses** filters, thins, removes poisons, toxins, excess protein, fat, cholesterol, uric acid, etc. and releases the blood.

- **Transforms** excess protein and fat (lipids) into cholesterol and lipoproteins (regulate cholesterol).

- **Transforms** poisons, toxins into bile, cholesterol, lecithin and other substances; cholesterol is broken down into bile salts and eliminated via the bowels.

Too much protein, fat, especially animal and fried foods thicken the blood too much, which in turn, thickens clogs and weakens the liver. Less protein, fat, cholesterol, uric acid, etc. are removed, more stays, **thickens the blood** (clots, high cholesterol and uric acid)

Too much animal protein causes excess clotting (thickening) of the blood. The clotting factor is protein based.

- **Blood clots** (thrombus)

All animal food contains saturated fat. **Saturated fat** (oily, greasy, high-energy source) contains cholesterol (essential part, fatty of every cell, tissue, especially brain and nerves). **Too much saturated fat** increases

- Blood **cholesterol**
- Low-density lipoproteins (**LDL**)
- Very low-density lipoproteins (**VLDL**)
- LDL and VLDL harden cholesterol into plaque
- **Plaque** pastes, narrows and clogs the arteries

Too much plaque and **clots**
- Paste, narrow, **clog** (atherosclerosis) and or **block** (occlude) the arteries decreasing size, diameter through which blood flows

Clogged arteries in the extreme

- Reduce blood, circulation to the extremities: head, arms and legs: arthritis, pain, inflammation, weakness, dryness, tension (chest) numbness and shaking, trembling (air, wind, vata)

- Darken, purple the complexion, lips, nails and skin (spider, varicose veins) in the arms, legs

- Cause a buildup and backflow of blood, energy heat: blood pressure, fever, higher body temperature, red skin, eyes, dizziness, headaches, insomnia

- Weakens, dries and inflames the **brain, nerves** (insomnia, shingles), etc.

- Smoking also dries constricts and narrows the arteries, worsens atherosclerosis, reducing blood flow, especially in the chest and arms

Too much animal protein, fat, in the extreme, also

- **Thickens, hardens the blood** into **cysts, lumps** (benign, harmless) and **tumors** (benign and malignant). Tumors (stagnant blood) overtime deteriorate, ferment, become **cancerous** (fixed in location, very painful) and or bleed, into the skin, stools, urine, etc.

- Thickens, darkens and clots menstrual blood causing painful menses, dysmenorrhea, endometriosis, tumors and or cancer.

- Thickens, inflames the **skin** (acne, warts, psoriasis, itching).

- Thickens, overheats the body, causes excessive perspiration via excess weight, insulation

Too much protein, fat and starch (processed grain)

- Clogs and over stimulates the **stomach**, hydrochloric acid (HCl): nausea, heartburn

- Clogs, overheats, dries, fouls the **large intestine**: dry stools, constipation, foul odor, tumors, cancer

The colder middle diet (54- 55), bitter herbs, less animal, more fruit, vegetables, beans, nuts (less), seeds, dairy, mild spices and bitter herbs (helps dissolve excess protein, fat, cholesterol, uric acid, plaque, etc.) is recommended for all high protein, fat diseases, in addition to medical consultation and or treatment.

Nuts, seeds and beans are high in **unsaturated fat** and high-density lipoproteins (**HDL**), which lower blood cholesterol, as does eating lesser animal otherwise history repeats itself. Too much lowers HDL.

60% of the diet should be vegetables (3- 5 per meal), 30% lightly cooked (broccoli, carrots, cauliflower, kale, squash, etc.) and 70% raw (beets, cabbage, celery, lettuce, etc.) and fruit (one per meal). Fruits and vegetables (water, enzymes, fiber, etc.) cleanse, cool and moisten the body.

Decrease dairy, nuts, grains, oil, fruit and juices if hot, damp (acne, rashes, psoriasis, etc.) kapha (page 42). Experiment and see what works, what does not. Severity of condition will determine the overall strictness of diet. Expand the diet (chicken, turkey) when necessary.

The body requires a certain amount or protein, fat. **Too little** thins, weakens the blood. Thin (low protein, low fat) blood (blood deficiency) weakens, thins all structure function.

Thin deficient blood, in the extreme

- Weakens, shortens or stops the menses: amenorrhea (little or no period), infertility miscarriage, short term pregnancy

- Causes hot flashes (blood is moistening, cooling).

- Weakens, dries, cracks and pales the skin, hair, nails, face, tongue, lips muscles, bones, brain, eyes, secretions, etc. Blood (red), protein, fat, builds, thickens, fuels, moistens.

- Dries and weakens the ligaments, tendons, muscles, nerves, causing pain, numbness, inflammation, shaking, tremors, arthritis, etc. in the arms, legs, hands and feet.

- Decreases circulation, blood, cools, dampens, dries the body, lowers body temperature, coldness

Thin, deficient blood (low protein, low fat),

- Cause insomnia. The spirit (consciousness) sleeps in the heart. Blood, protein, fat or jing deficiency weakens the heart's ability to hold the spirit, making it hard to fall and stay asleep.

- Dry and weaken the brain cause dizziness swaying and or loss of consciousness. A lack of blood causes a lack of holding. Smoking, caffeine and alcohol worsen.

- Dry and weakens the brain, nerves, reducing ability to focus, remember, hold thoughts, etc.

- Cause Attention Deficit Disorder (ADD), senility, irrationality, and or hysteria (men and women)

- Cause **Alzheimer** disease. The brain, nerves are blood, protein and fat rich. Many patients when autopsied have dry, gray brains instead of moist, red, indicating decreased blood flow via blood deficiency and or clogged arteries.

- Thin, break down tumors, cholesterol, plaque

The hotter middle diet (page 56- 57) is recommended for cold, deficient dietary diseases.

Body fluids moisten the skin, muscles, joints (synovial fluids), spine, organs and the orifices of the eyes, ears, nose and mouth with tears, wax, mucous and saliva, and help form urine and gastric juices. Too much or too little fluid tends to cause disease.

Body temperature (98.6°F), spices (hot) and digestion regulate, heat, dry and thin bodily fluids.

Colder temperatures via cold, damp climate or diet weaken digestion, decrease nutrient absorption, blood, body temperature, which cools, thickens fluids into

- Mucous, phlegm
- Cysts, edema
- Vaginal discharges, yeast infections

Too many salads, juices, cold drinks, especially at the beginning of the meal, in the extreme, cools, dampens, decreases digestion, nutrient absorption, blood, energy, body temperature.

Grains, especially processed (bread, noodles, cookies, pretzels, chips, etc.) are also damp, moistening. Too many tends to cause excessive dampness, paste in the intestines, which in turn, causes abdominal bloating, gas, offensive, sweet body odor and or bad breath (**halitosis**).

Cooked foods and spices (page 73- 75) heat dry and drain dampness, "wet" conditions of the body.

Body fluids excess
- Mucus, phlegm (white, clear), pleurisy
- Swollen hands, feet, edema (arms, legs, ankles)
- Cellulite, copious, clear urination, bladder infections, cysts and or stones, tendency to cry

Phlegm (thick mucous)
- Harden into cysts, stones
- Cause bone deformities: rheumatoid arthritis
- Lodge in the lungs: coughing, sleep apnea
- Lodge in the breasts: cysts, fibrocystic
- Lodge in the heart: mental confusion
- Lodge in the gall bladder: kidneys cysts, stones
- Lodge in the head: slurred speech, incoherence
- Takes weeks, months to dissolve

Too little fluid via blood deficiency, hemorrhage, excessive sweating, purging (vomiting, diarrhea, laxatives) and sex tends to cause dryness: respiration (dry cough, sore throat), elimination (dry stools, constipation), skin (dry, itching). Too much heat and dryness via climate, smoking, alcohol, hot spices and fried foods, tends to cause dryness. Caffeine in any form is very drying. It also drains consumes jing.

Deficient body fluids dry, vata

- Dry skin, mouth, nose, throat, lungs, itching
- Coughing, sinusitis, scanty urination, dry stools
- Constipation
- Stiff, tight joints, muscles, tendons, ligaments

7

Spleen

Food → digestion→ **blood** → structure→ function

The spleen (large oval organ attached to the pancreas) is located on the left side of the body between the stomach (paired organ) and diaphragm.

- **Controls digestion, pancreas, stomach**
- **Controls blood**
- **Controls chi** energy, function (blood fuels chi)
- **Origin of damp** (digestion heats, dries the body)

Digestion breaks down, separates food into nutrients and non-nutrients. Nutrients are transported into blood. **Blood** (watery medium) transports nutrients, hormones, wastes, etc. to and from every cell, tissue, structure, function. All food, nutrients and non-nutrients, not digested absorbed is waste and moved down into the large intestine for eventual elimination.

TCM: Spleen yang provides the **fire** that cooks food and fluids inside the stomach and small intestine, separating the pure (nutrients) from the impure (fiber, non-nutrients) essences.

The pure essences, nutrients mist, rise up (via spleen yang) into the lungs, and combine with the pure essences of air (oxygen) before moving down into the heart for the final transformation into blood. Kidney yang fuels all yang (function).

The **stomach** is the first and strongest stage of digestion. It produces hydrochloric acid (**HCl**) and other enzymes specifically designed to digest animal protein, fat. The second stage occurs in the small intestine.

The **small intestine** (22") receives enzymes and bile from the **pancreas** and **liver** via pancreatic and gall bladder ducts. Pancreatic enzymes digest protein, fat and sugar into smaller, more absorbable sizes. Bile (fat emulsifier) breaks down fat. Nutrients are absorbed directly into the bloodstream, lymph via villi and lacteals in the small intestine.

The quality and quantity of food, nutrients determine digestion, blood and all structure function. Protein and fat build, fuel, heat all structure function. Fruits, vegetables, water, minerals etc. reduce, cleanse, cool and moisten.

- **Too much** protein, fat and grain pastes, clogs and weakens the stomach and intestines, reducing digestion, nutrient absorption, blood and elimination.

- **Too little protein, fat** reduces digestion, nutrient absorption, blood, elimination, energy, etc.

- **Too many cold, damp** foods (milk, ice cream), drinks (juices, soda, ice water) dilute digestive acids, enzymes, reducing digestion, nutrient absorption, blood, energy, body temperature, etc.

Digestion (three meals per day) also heats the body. Normal **body temperature** (98.6°F) heats, dries and thins bodily fluids. Lower, colder body temperatures cool, harden, thicken and slow bodily fluids, in the same way the colder temperatures of night and winter cool, harden water in the air and on the ground into the morning dew, rain, snow and or ice.

Lower, colder body temperatures via cold, damp (wet) diet, climate (winter, air conditioning, etc.) or chronic illness, thicken and harden bodily fluids in the lungs, throat sinuses, breasts, vagina and uterus

- Mucous, phlegm, cysts
- Coughing, snoring, sleep apnea
- Shortness of breath, asthma
- Vaginal discharge, yeast infection

In TCM, **the spleen is the origin of dampness, and the lungs its receptacle**. Digestive energy, spleen yang, fire rises up into the lungs, and spreads, moves down into sexual organs below. Weak digestion (cold spleen) provides less fire, heat, which increases cold, lower body temperatures and dampness.

Low protein, low fat (especially soft dairy) and high carbohydrate (fruits, juices, sugar and cold drinks) diet weaken, cool digestion as does excessive sex.

Sex, orgasm, blood, protein and deficiency, and **caffeine** decreases jing. Jing (sexual essence) powers all structure function. **Jing depletion** weakens and cools all structure, function.

The sun, protein, fat, **hot spices** (cardamom, basil, cayenne, black pepper, turmeric, ginger, etc.) and exercise stimulate digestion, heat the body, dry fluids.

Weak digestion tends to attack women and children more than men. Many women tend to have weak digestion via menstruation and the tendency to eat too many **cold, damp** foods: milk, yogurt, cottage cheese and ice cream, salads, fruits, juices, smoothies, shakes, cold drinks, etc. Menstruation, blood loss temporarily weakens cools all function.

Children (underdeveloped) tend to suffer from indigestion (abdominal bloating, gas, etc.) especially when eating a cold, damp diet (milk and cereal, ice cream, tropical fruits, juices, cold drinks, soda and sugar).

Milk and cereal is very difficult to digest, as milk tends to curdle, enclose grains, forming a protective barrier where digestive enzymes cannot fully penetrate. Partially digested food becomes waste product, paste that builds, accumulates in the intestines, further inhibiting, reducing digestion, nutrient absorption, blood and elimination. Cardamom and ginger aid in the digestion of dairy.

Men are the opposite. They tend to have stronger digestion, higher metabolism via testosterone (hot, fiery hormone) and the tendency to eat high protein, high fat diets, which is why men rarely suffer from excess water weight, edema, although too much too much protein, fat and starch, will cause indigestion.

The spleen controls digestion. Digestion controls blood. Blood (nutrients) controls every structure, function (chi, yang). There are **four major pathologies** associated with the spleen.

Stage 1. Spleen chi deficiency weak digestion

- Slows the movement of food, causing it to collect within the stomach and small intestine, **bloating**, distending the abdomen

- Causes **gas, flatulence burping** and or **loose stools**. Spices (73) aid digestion; help counter gas, flatulence, burping, bloating, loose stools (watery).

Stage 2. Blood deficiency

Weak digestion decreases nutrient absorption, thins the blood, decreases circulation, tends to cause:

- **Coldness** as less blood, protein and fat produces less energy, heat, colder body temperatures.

- **Sallow complexion**, pale, dry tongue, weakness, inflammation pain, numbness, shaking, etc. as less blood (red, moist, etc.) is circulated.

- **Weak appetite**. It takes energy, blood, protein and fat to stimulate, fuel appetite.

Stage 3. Spleen yang deficiency

Chronically weak digestion (spleen yang) tends to

- Cause loose stools with undigested food and or chronic diarrhea (parasites, bacteria also a cause)

- Increase waste product, excess weight, heaviness and a subsequent bearing down, heavy sensation, excess heat in the intestines.

- **Cool and moisten** the lungs, nose throat, ears (inner ear infection, loss of hearing) and sexual organs with excess fluids: mucous, phlegm, white vaginal discharges (leucorrhea).

- Increase stomach fluids causing them to overflow onto the tongue creating a moist, thick, clear or white coating, Clear and white are the colors of cold (rain, ice and snow). A normal, healthy tongue is pink with a slight coating.

- **Food allergies**. Clogged intestines tend to cause weak, incomplete digestion of normally easy to digest foods (fruits, vegetables and grains) that suddenly become difficult to digest, resulting in food allergies. Strengthening the digestive organs via proper diet and herbs is the best way to clean the intestines, strengthen digestion, and or cure food allergies, although some food allergies may not correct via diet.

Stage 4. Chronic blood deficiency tends to

- Easily bruise and bleed the skin, capillaries. Tumors and stones (kidney, bladder) also cause blood in the urine, stools.

- Cause bright, white (color of cold) complexion.

- Dry, weaken, shake and tremble the arms, legs, bones, ligaments, muscles, etc.

- Cool, weaken, slow the body (via less blood, energy), which in turn, can depress the mind. Modern medicine normally treats depression with amphetamines, stimulants drugs (heat, move fluids, food, emotions, etc.). Hot soups, spices, sunshine, exercise also heat and move.

- Weaken, drain organ chi (stomach, uterus, rectum, etc.) causing them to sink, prolapse. Spleen chi, yang ascends, lifts, and holds organs, blood, etc. in their place. Chronic blood deficiency weakens the spleen, holding.

The hotter middle diet, meal plan (pages 56- 57) is recommended for all cold, damp, deficient conditions.

Too much animal protein, fat, and starch tend to cause heartburn, nausea, acid regurgitation, pain, stomach ulcers, pancreatitis and or tumors.

The spleen and brain have an intimate relationship as both separate the pure from impure.

- The spleen, digestion separates the pure food essences (nutrients) from the impure (non-nutrients, preservatives, etc.).

- The brain separates pure, relevant thoughts, stimuli, from the impure, irrelevant.

Good diet and strong digestion strengthens, purifies the blood, which in turn, strengthens, increases the brain's ability to separate, think clearly, analyze, remember, etc. Weak digestion, overeating, etc. clouds, confuses the mind.

In TCM, the **pancreas** is part of the spleen. The pancreas produces digestive enzymes and regulates blood sugar via the production of insulin and glucagon. Insulin lowers the level of blood sugar (glucose) by converting it into glycogen (storage form of glucose), which is stored in the liver and muscles. Low blood sugar causes the pancreas secretes glucagon, which converts glycogen in the liver into glucose, released back into the bloodstream, raising blood sugar.

The pancreas and liver control the level of blood sugar. The correct amount produces health. Too much sugar or too much insulin tends to cause hyperglycemia. Too little sugar or insulin tends to cause hypoglycemia and or diabetes. **There are two kinds of diabetes**: diabetes insipidus and diabetes mellitus.

Diabetes mellitus (more common) is a chronic, complex metabolic disorder due to partial or total lack of insulin or the inability of insulin to function normally causing excessive urination, thirst, weight loss and excessive sugar in the blood or urine.

Diabetes is common with age. Adult onset diabetes, depending upon severity is generally curable through diet, discipline. Juvenile diabetes is more difficult to treat, cure, as it tends to be genetically predisposed, attacking during childhood.

In TCM

- **Sweet taste** (sugar, fruits, vegetables, grain, meat, chicken, Siberian ginseng, etc) stimulates the spleen, pancreas. Too many sweet foods over stimulates and weakens the spleen, pancreas, liver, digestion, blood sugar, etc. Cooked food and spices help digest and eliminate sugar.

- **Yellow, orange** colored foods (carrots, hard squashes, etc.) nourish the spleen

The spleen, pancreas and stomach (paired organs) and small intestine control digestion and are highly charged, at their energetic peak, in the early morning and afternoon, and weakest, at night, which is why big (protein, fat) breakfast, big lunch and small dinner are often advised. You are not only what you eat, but also what you digest or not digest.

- **Stomach** 7:00 A.M. - 9:00 A.M.
- **Spleen** 9:00 A.M. - 11:00 A.M.
- **Heart** 11:00 A.M. - 1:00 P.M.
- **Small Intestine** 1:00 P.M. - 3:00 P.M

8

Stomach and Small Intestine

Digestion and absorption occur in the stomach and small intestine. Spleen yang (chi) provides the fire that cooks food and fluids inside the stomach and small intestine, separating the pure (nutrients) from the impure food essences (non-nutrients, fiber, etc.). The pure essences are "misted up" via spleen yang to the lungs, to combine with the pure essences of air (oxygen) and sent down into the heart for the final transformation into blood. All food, nutrients, etc. not digested, absorbed becomes waste (large intestine).

The stomach mixes food and fluids with **hydrochloric acid (HCl)** and other enzymes specifically designed to digest animal protein, fat (saturated), which is harder, more difficult to digest, eliminate than plant (nuts, seeds) fat. Food, fluid and acid, sit, mix, **ferment (sour)**, break apart in the stomach before moving down (stomach chi descends) via the pylorus (end, tubular portion of stomach, encircled by pyloric sphincter) into the duodenum (first section small intestine)

Overeating, especially protein, fat and flour, late meals, snacks or lying down after meals tends to clog, obstruct the stomach and small intestine, cause a rebellion, back flow, of energy, heat (like a clogged, overflowing drain)

- Burping, nausea, vomiting or sour body odor

Chronic overeating, especially protein, fat and starch over stimulates the stomach, production of HCL, in the extreme, cause **burning** of the stomach's lining (**ulcers**). Raw celery and lettuce help relieve burning. Preventative-cayenne pepper (in vegetable soup) irritates stimulates the lining of the stomach causing it to secrete mucous (protective covering of the lining). Bitter herbs also help. Check with your doctor. Too much protein, fat, also forms polyps and tumors.

Chronically weak digestion and too many sour foods (dairy) tend to cause **sour body odor**, breath. Food that remains in the stomach, too long, tends to over-ferment, sour, causing an excessive sour smell, that rises, moves up and out the throat, breath and skin. Too many cold drinks, salads, juices, overeating, tight clothing, etc. decrease stomach energy, downward movement of food, allowing it to collect, ferment. Cooked foods and spices increase digestion.

The small intestine (22 feet) receives predigested food from the stomach, and **bile** (fat emulsifier) and **pancreatic enzymes** from the *liver* and pancreas via *gall bladder* and pancreatic ducts. Bile is stored in the gall bladder prior to its release into the small intestine. Digestion (separation of pure and impure) occurs primarily in the small intestine. The pure (nutrients) are absorbed through the villi (fingerlike projections extending from the inner walls of the small intestine) and lacteals into the bloodstream.

The villi contain capillaries (connected to arterioles, arteries and venules, veins) and lacteals (lymph channels that absorb digested fat). Absorption of nutrients decreases when excess food debris clogs, pastes the villi. Bitter herbs increase digestion and absorption in the small intestine.

Processed grains (noodles, bread, cookies, etc.), protein, fat and oil are thick, gooey, sticky, and tend to clog and paste the villi, walls of the small intestine:

- Painful, hard abdominal bloating, heartburn, etc. sometimes diagnosed as digestive allergies

Raw vegetables and fruits (high fiber content) act like a broom in sweeping the intestines clean of any excess food debris. **Too many** fruits, juices, cold drinks weaken digestion, decrease nutrient absorption, moisten, loosen the stools while increasing urination.

The small intestine also digests and distills fluids into pure and impure. The pure transform into body fluids (humors): mucous, tears, synovial (lubricate the joints). The impure fluids move down to the large intestine.

Small intestine symptoms

- Excessive appetite, abdominal pain caused by food stagnation, flatulence (offensive sweet or sour smell), borborygmus (stomach gurgling)

- Pale copious urine (cold condenses), scanty dark urine (excess heat dries, burns), dry stools (excess heat) and or vomiting

- Bleeding gums the stomach and large intestine meridians (energetic pathways) pass through the mouth, gums. Overeating can adversely affect, overheat, swell the stomach and large intestine, causing the gums to bleed, as can poor diet, poor dental hygiene and or smoking (receding gums).

The body, according to TCM has a daily cycle of energy.

There are 24 hours in a day and 12 major organs. Each organ has a two-hour period, when it is highly charged. Digestive organs are highly charged between the hours of 7 A.M. and 3 P.M., which is why the heaviest foods, nutrients (protein, and fat) are generally eaten for breakfast and lunch. Digestion is weakest during the evening. Eat a small dinner.

Daily cycle of energy

- Stomach 7:00 A.M. - 9:00 A.M.
- Spleen 9:00 A.M. - 11:00 A.M.
- Heart 11:00 A.M. - 1:00 P.M.
- Small Intestine 1:00 P.M. - 3:00 P.M

To improve digestion, elimination

- Eat from hot (building) to cold (cleansing).
- Eat more (protein, fat) during the day.
- Eat 3-5 vegetables (cooked, raw) with spices and or oil and 1 fruit per meal.
- Eat 1 plate of food per meal (quantity spoils quality).
- Eat while sitting down. Wear loose comfortable clothing. Do not lie down after eating.
- Take a short walk after a meal.

9

Large Intestine & Urinary Bladder

The large intestine (5') and urinary bladder, located in the lower abdomen, store and eliminate waste products (feces and urine). They are largely a function of diet.

The small intestine (tube) connects to the large intestine (tube). Food, nutrients and non-nutrients (includes fiber) not digested, absorbed in the small intestine becomes waste that passes → **large intestine → (1) cecum** (beginning sac, in lower right abdomen, contains appendix, offshoot of cecum)→ **(2) ascending→ (3) transverse→ (4) descending colon→ (5) rectum.**

The stools are made from food, nutrients and non-nutrients. Protein, fat and starch paste, harden the stools and intestines. Fruits and vegetables loosen and bulk the stools.

High protein, fat (especially animal) and starch (processed grains) diets, overeating, big dinners, late night snacks, obesity, sleeping late and sedentary lifestyle tends to cause

- Gas, painful bloating
- Dry or pasty stools, foul odor
- Constipation (difficult or infrequent elimination)
- Pain, pressure in rectum, anus
- Pockets (diverticulitis), polyps, tumors, cancer
- Ulcers (ulcerative colitis)

Vegetables and fruits liquefy, soften and thin the stools. **Too many** fruits, juices, cold drinks, **sugar** loosen the stools and decrease elimination. Too little dries, constipates the stools. Normal, healthy stools are firm and relatively odorless.

Fiber found in vegetables, fruits and psyllium husks swell with water, which in turn swells, adds bulk to the stools, making them easy to pass.

The large intestine is energetically active from 5:00 A.M. to 7:00 A.M. It is common, healthy to move the bowels during this time. If you eat 2- 3 meals a day, you should move your bowels two to three times a day, especially in the A.M.

For hot, yang (high protein, high fat) constipation, the colder middle diet is recommended in addition to

- Black fungus
- 1TB of sesame or olive oil (1- 2X/ day with food),
- Aloe vera gel (laxative) in juice and or psyllium husks 1-2 TB in 1-2 glasses of water, twice daily
- Smaller, earlier meals
- Drinking fruit juice or cold water or exercising after awakening helps move the bowels.
- Take a short walk after a meal.
- Alternately contracting and relaxing the anal sphincter muscles helps relieve anal, rectal pain
- Enemas, colonics and laxatives may help but not cure chronic constipation, as they do not remove the cause: poor diet, lifestyle, which grows the disease. Long-term use increases constipation.

All waste products, especially animal putrefy. Daily elimination is necessary; otherwise, re-absorption of poisons into the blood, lymph can occur.

Long-term constipation (difficult or infrequent elimination) increases the chance of re-absorption, autointoxication and eventual weakening of the immune system, producing antibodies that attack healthy tissues. The large intestine tends to be the breeding ground, not the cause of autoimmune illnesses. Most autoimmune diseases share similar *symptoms, diets.*

Lupus: *abdominal pain*, weight loss, fatigue, skin rash, *nausea, vomiting, diarrhea* and *constipation*

Crohn's Disease: *pain* in abdomen, right lower quadrant, appendix, *diarrhea, nausea,* fever, *fatigue*, weight loss

Fibromyalgia: chronic, achy muscular *pain*, dizziness, *fatigue*, Irritable Bowel Syndrome, CFS

Chronic Fatigue Syndrome (CFS): *extreme fatigue*, aching muscles, joints, headaches, low blood pressure, fever, loss of appetite, upper respiratory infections, nasal congestion, mucous, phlegm, Candidiasis, *loose stools, diarrhea, constipation,* depression, anxiety, etc.

Irritable Bowel Syndrome (IBS): *abdominal pain*, gas, bloating, cramps, *loose stools, diarrhea, constipation*

All disease progresses in stages. Stage 1 is cause

- **(1) Poor diet** weakens, sickens
- **(2) Digestion** bloating, gas, nausea, pain
- **(3) Elimination** loose stools, constipation
- **(4) Blood** fatigue, pallor
- **(5) Circulation** coldness, inflammation
- **(6) Organ function** autoimmune disease

The lungs and large intestine are paired organs (TCM). Exercise stimulates the breath, expansion and contraction of the lungs, which moves the **diaphragm** (muscular partition, divides chest and abdomen).

As the diaphragm moves, up and down, it massages the small intestine increasing peristalsis.

Peristalsis is the wavelike contractions of the smooth muscle of the digestive tract that fosters downward movement of food and fluids, urination and defecation. Most athletes and active people in general do not suffer constipation. They also tend to eat well.

The **urinary bladder** (sac) stores and eliminates urine received from the kidneys. The kidneys filter the blood remove wastes, especially **nitrogen**, urea, mixes with water in urine that passes into the bladder via ureters (connecting tubes), eventually eliminated via the urethra (hollow tube). Kidney yang (fire) heats, thins the urine in the bladder making it easy to pass. Deficient kidney yang thickens and slows fluids.

Too many cold, damp foods (ice cream, salads, tropical fruits, juices and cold drinks) tend to thicken (and cloud) the urine making it frequent, sticky, difficult and or painful to pass. Too much water in the extreme, overworks the kidneys, bladder (excessive urination, edema). Drinking eight glasses of water per day may be good for some, but not necessarily all. Anything can be done to extreme, excess or deficiency.

The hotter middle diet, cranberry juice and bitter herbs are recommended for cold, damp bladder infections. (More info pages 285- 287)

Excessive heat, dampness (animal, fried foods, alcohol and hot spices) tends to dry, burn, thicken and darken (turbid) the urine (sand, stones) making it frequent, painful and smelly.

10

Liver and Gall Bladder

Food→ digestion→ **blood**→ structure→ function →

The liver (body's largest organ) and gall bladder (paired organ) are located in the upper right part of the abdominal cavity, rib cage. All blood passes through the liver. **The liver stores, cleanses, transforms and releases the blood**

- **Cleanses** filters, thins, removes poisons, toxins, excess protein, fat, cholesterol, uric acid, etc.

- **Transforms** excess fat and protein into cholesterol and lipoproteins (regulate cholesterol)

- **Transforms** poisons, toxins into bile, cholesterol, lecithin and other substances

- **Bile** (fat emulsifier, digests, breaks down fat) is stored in the gall bladder and later released via bile duct into the duodenum, small intestine.

- **Releases**, distributes cleansed blood (nutrients) that nourish all structure function. Regular cleansing and distribution of the blood insures the **smooth the flow of chi.** Blocked, trapped blood, chi in the liver tends to cause abdominal swelling, right-sided pain, irritability and anger.

The heart (pump) commands, controls the **circulation of blood** via its system of vessels.

Arteries (except pulmonary) carry oxygen-enriched blood away from the heart. **Veins** (except pulmonary) carry de-oxygenated blood to the heart. Smaller branches of arteries (arterioles) and veins (venules) connect to capillaries. **Capillaries** connect to all tissue passing nutrients, absorbing wastes through thin, porous walls.

The quality and quantity of food, nutrients, and exercise determines the overall quality, quantity of blood, circulation and all structure function. Building nutrients: protein and fat (saturated and unsaturated), foods **thicken** the blood. Cleansing nutrients, foods, thin.

Animal foods (red meat, chicken, turkey, eggs, and hard cheese) are high in protein, saturated fat. A certain amount of animal protein and saturated fat is beneficial, healthy, especially for deficiency and cold climates.

Too much protein thickens the blood too much forming **clots** (thrombus)

Saturated fat, high in **cholesterol** (essential part of every cell, tissue, especially the brain, nerves); increases (1) blood cholesterol, (2) low-density (LDL) and (3) very low-density (VLDL) lipoproteins. **LDL** and **VLDL** harden cholesterol into **plaque** (thick, sticky). Excess plaque pastes, narrows (atherosclerosis) and or blocks the arteries reducing circulation, nutrient absorption and waste exchange, especially in the extremities: head, arms and legs causing fatigue, pain, dizziness, insomnia, arthritis, dryness, inflammation, shaking, etc.

Unsaturated fat found in beans, nuts and seeds increase the number of high-density lipoproteins (HDL). Too much lowers. **HDL removes and transports cholesterol** back to the liver, where it is broken down and transformed into bile salts, eliminated in the bowels

All blood passes through the liver. The liver stores, cleanses, thins and releases the blood. **Too much protein, fat** especially animal, thickens clogs and weakens the liver. Less protein, fat, uric acid, etc. are cleansed, removed more stays in the

- Blood (clots, high cholesterol, uric acid)
- Arteries (plaque, atherosclerosis)
- Joints (gout)
- Skin (acne, psoriasis, warts)

Clogged, narrow arteries (atherosclerosis) and swollen liver reduce circulation, blood flow (nutrients, waste exchange) especially to the extremities (head, arms and legs) producing quasi blood deficiency symptoms (fatigue, dryness, inflammation, coldness, etc.) in addition to excess heat.

Clogged fatty, hardened liver tends to

- Enlarge, swell with blood as more blood passes in than out, decreasing circulation, especially to the head, arms and legs causing moodiness, irritability, muscular tension, pain, etc.

- Press out distend the ribs, upper abdomen, chest, breasts cause difficulty swallowing, imaginary lump in throat, (plum pit syndrome).

- Cause sighing: body, lung's attempt to release trapped energy (chi) and blood within the liver. The lungs (right lung sits atop the liver) expand and contract, which in turn massages and helps move blood in and out of the liver.

- Weaken, thicken the blood (clots, high cholesterol) and clog, narrow and harden the arteries.

Thick blood and clogged arteries tend to

- Reduce circulation, blood (nutrient flow to the arms and legs: fatigue, pain, dryness, inflammation, numbness, arthritis, etc,

- Darken and clot menstrual blood, cause PMS and or dysmenorrhea (painful or irregular periods). Thick high protein, fat liver blood passes directly and unevenly into the uterus.

- Cause high blood pressure, red face, eyes, skin (heat rises, moves blood up, out, reddens head, skin), purple lips, excessive thinking, dreaming, wakefulness (insomnia) or loud ringing in the ears (tinnitus). Sleeping is a cooling, calming activity. Overeating, obesity and anger overheat the body.

- Reduce blood, nutrient flow to the head, dizziness, poor vision, weak hearing, damaging, drying, thinning, cracking or bleeding the capillaries in the nose, nosebleeds (epitasis)

- Reduce blood, nutrient flow to the brain causing it to shrink, dry, harden and or short-circuit aneurism, dementia and Alzheimer's disease (long-term blood deficiency is also a cause).

The liver removes poisons, toxins from the blood and transforms them into bile, cholesterol, lecithin and other substances. One pint of bile per day passes into the gall bladder and later released into small intestine (via cystic and bile ducts), eventually passing into the feces. Abnormal concentration of bile (yellow) acids, cholesterol and phospholipids in the bile tend to create stones in the gall bladder, ducts. Excess bile, in the extreme can leak, overflow into the skin, yellowing the skin, eyes (jaundice).

Long-term high protein, fat diets (increase bile production) tend to cause gallstones, which can collect, stay in place or move, travel into the bile ducts causing inflammation, nausea, vomiting, fever and or pain in the right upper abdomen or behind the breastbone.

Gall bladder attacks (mimic heart attack pain), high among men (high protein, fat and starch diets) tend to occur after fried, fatty meals, in the extreme, clogging the stomach and small intestine causing a backflow (rebellion) of stomach energy, food and bile: burping, nausea, vomiting acid, bile or bitter taste.

The colder middle diet, spices (cumin, coriander and fennel), bitter herbs (page 54- 55) and occasional fasting is recommended for all high protein, fat, pitta diseases (hyperactive, swollen liver). **Reduce** pungent (hot spices), sour and salty foods, herbs, which aggravate high protein, fat, yang, pitta diseases.

Bitter herbs: golden seal, barberry, gentian and turmeric one capsule, or 10- 20 drops (alcohol or non-alcohol tincture) each of in hot water (let sit few minutes, dissipates alcohol, increases absorption) can be taken one to two times per day for 1- 2 weeks or more. **Aloe vera gel** (2- 3 ounces) in fruit juice (apple, orange) 2- 3 times per day also helps cool, thin and detoxify the liver (swollen) and spleen. Too much bitter tends to cause headaches and nausea. **Radishes and apple cider vinegar** (1 TB in one glass of water, three times per day) may help dissolve gallstones, in addition to dietary changes. Consult with a physician.

Peppermint tea cools, relaxes liver (and muscle) tension. Fish liver oil supplements may aggravate, worsen and tighten the liver, as can anger.

Coffee enemas also help detoxify the liver. For more information please read **A Cancer Therapy, Results of Fifty Cases** by Max Garson, M.D. Check with your doctor first.

Blood, protein and fat deficiency can also attack and weaken the liver. Liver blood nourishes the nails, eyes, sinews (tendons, ligaments) and uterus. Liver blood deficiency tends to cause dry nails, eyes, tendons, and amenorrhea (little or no period).

Blood, protein and fat deficiency is generally easy but time-consuming (120 days) to rebuild, cure. The hotter middle diet (page 56) is recommended for blood deficiency, caused by low protein, low fat diets. Protein and fat are easier to digest, absorb and eliminate when cooked with vegetables in soups, stews.

In TCM
- **Sour taste** (lemons, yogurt, sauerkraut, fermented foods, etc.) heats, stimulates the liver, increases secretion of bile, which **benefits** a deficient liver, blood conditions, but will aggravate, tighten a clogged, fatty, swollen liver and spleen (excess heat, yang, pitta), and is therefore avoided
- **Green color** soothes the liver. Green vegetables (broccoli, cabbage, kale and collards), chlorophyll, etc. cool, cleanse, break down and eliminate excess protein, fat, paste and toxins.
- **Sides of the tongue** represent the liver and gall bladder. Liver, gallbladder heat via long-term high protein, fat, diets, alcohol and smoking tend to dry, redden and or yellow the tongue's coating or sides.
- **A vertical line between the eyebrows** generally indicates liver congestion. Two to three vertical lines indicate gall bladder congestion (fat).

11

Heart

The heart is located in the chest, left center between the lungs and divided into left and right sides by a septum, upper (**atrium**) and lower (**ventricle**) chambers. Deoxygenated blood from the upper half of the body flows via the **Superior vena cava** (major vein) into the heart, **right** side→ right atrium→ right ventricle→ pulmonary artery→ lungs. The lungs cleanse, oxygenate and return the blood via the pulmonary vein→ **left** side of the heart→ left atrium→ left ventricle→ aorta→ to the rest of body.

→ Arteries

Food→ digestion→ **Blood**   → Capillaries→

→ Veins

(1) The heart **commands the blood.** Blood (watery medium) carries nutrients, hormones, wastes, etc. to from every cell, tissue) and **blood vessels. Arteries** (except pulmonary) carry oxygen-enriched blood away from the heart. **Veins** (except pulmonary) carry de-oxygenated blood to the heart. Smaller branches of arteries (arterioles) and veins (venules) connect to capillaries. **Capillaries** connect to all tissues, structure functions, passing nutrients and receiving, absorbing wastes through thin, one-cell layer thick walls. The complete circuit of blood, head to toe and back, occurs once every ninety seconds. The heart never stops beating, pumping generally 60- 80 times per minute.

The quality and quantity of **food, nutrients**, and exercise determines the overall quality, quantity of blood, circulation and all structure function.

Protein and fat are thick, hard, sticky nutrients.

- Too much thickens the blood and clogs the arteries, reducing circulation, nutrient and waste exchange, especially in the extremities: head, arms and legs.

- Too little thins, weakens, dries, inflames, while also reducing circulation, nutrient and waste exchange.

The following are **heart-related blood deficiency symptoms**

- Decreased circulation, blood, nutrient and waste exchange especially to the extremities causing coldness, fatigue, pain, inflammation, numbness

- Discomfort, dryness, tension and pain in the chest region as deficient, thin blood dries the sinews, muscles, tendons, etc. restricting movement, expansion and contraction, causing pain.

- Pale, dull, thin dry face, lips, tongue (blood is red)

- Facial pallor, in the extreme, bright, **white** (symbol of coldness) complexion

- Lethargy, sluggishness, apathy, easily startled

- Light-headedness, dizziness, dementia, Alzheimer's disease (gray brain, blood deficient) caused by severe blood deficiency, lack of holding, physical and mental. The swaying of dizziness mimics the movement of fire (dryness and heat create wind).

- Poor memory, forgetfulness, confusion

- Shaking, tremors, paralysis, loss of consciousness classified as air, wind (TCM) and vata (Ayurveda)

- **Palpitations** (conscious awareness of an acute, rapid beating, fluttering of the heart via a sudden drop in blood, pressure), dizziness via chronic anemia, blood deficiency, clogged arteries, hemorrhage, emotional trauma, etc.

- Light fever, perspiration. Chronic blood deficiency fails to moisten, contain energy, heat, allowing it (heat, perspiration) to boil over in small amounts.

- **Aneurism** (see page 127)

- Pale, thin and dry tongue, skin and hair. The heart opens up, pours blood (red) into the tongue. A normal healthy tongue is pinkish red with a light white coating. It fits the mouth perfectly, neither too large nor too small. Blood deficiency creates a thin, dry and or pale tongue.

The heart also **stores the shen** (spirit mind). The spirit (consciousness, life force) resides in the brain and spine. During the day, sunshine, the spirit rises up into the head, brain, stimulating thinking. At night, it sinks down, into the heart and "sleeps", rejuvenating body mind and spirit as does love. Thin (deficient) blood (1) does not moisten, control fire, but instead dries and occasionally flashes the body, (2) weakens the heart's holding power, grasp, allowing the spirit to wander during the night rise up into the brain, stimulate thinking, dreaming , dream disturbed sleep, **insomnia**.

Blood, protein and fat deficiency tends to attack women (menstruation and tendency to low protein, low diet, predisposes them towards blood deficiency).

The **hotter middle diet** (page 56- 57) is recommended for blood, protein and fat deficiency.

Too much protein, fat tends to thicken the blood and arteries too much, while also weakening the liver. All blood passes through the liver. The liver stores, cleanses (removes excess protein, fat, cholesterol, etc.) and releases the blood. Too much protein, fat clogs and weakens the liver. Less protein, fat, cholesterol is removed, more stays (blood clots, high cholesterol).

Clots (**thrombus**) are fibrous blood (thickened by protein-based clotting factors) that travel independently or clump together with plaque and block, occlude a coronary artery causing a heart attack (**myocardial infarction**). Excess protein increases clotting just as excess cholesterol increases plaque.

Too much fat, cholesterol, in the extreme, thickens, clogs the arteries (**plaque, atherosclerosis**) reducing circulation, especially to head arms and legs. Once the blood and arteries saturate with excess protein, fat, a single meal, small portion of animal or fried foods, alcohol and or sugar (all excess sugar turns into fat) is enough to precipitate a clog, which can contract and or close an artery, reduce blood flow to the brain. The following are symptoms of **high protein, high fat blood** (clots, high cholesterol) attacking, **weakening the heart**, blood vessels, brain, etc.

- Clogged, narrow arteries (**atherosclerosis**)

- Reduced circulation, blood to the extremities: head, arms and legs, **arthritis**, pain (in the arms, legs, especially when sitting or lying down), inflammation, numbness

- **High blood pressure**, insomnia

- **Red** face, eyes, tongue (red body, points, ulcers)

- Increased heart rate (**tachycardia**)

- Burning sensation, constriction in the chest

- Nausea, **dizziness**, fainting

- Block, clog the coronary artery producing intense chest pain (**angina pectoris**) radiating down the left arm, cause shortness of breath, fainting, anxiety, sweating dizziness, seizures and or aneurism (may burst).

- **Headaches**, restlessness, agitation

- **Aneurism** is a saclike widening in a blood vessel), seizure, heart attack, cerebrovascular accident (stroke, paralysis) and or coma.

- Chronic atherosclerosis reduces circulation, blood to the head, brain, and in the extreme, dries the heart, nerves, muscles, etc. causing them to seize, contract, collapse, or die.

The colder middle diet (page 54), raw beets, berries, bitter herbs, cayenne pepper (helps prevent blood clots) and occasional fasting is recommended for all high protein, high fat, pitta diseases, in addition to medical consultation. **Bitter herbs:** 1 capsule, or 10- 20 drops (alcohol or non-alcohol tincture) each of **golden seal, barberry, gentian and turmeric** in hot water (let sit few minutes, dissipates alcohol) can be taken one to two times per day. **Aloe vera gel** (2- 3 ounces) in fruit juice (apple, orange) 2- 3 times per day also helps. Bitter herbs (cold, drying) detoxify, breakdown excess fat, cholesterol in the liver and spleen, stimulate the heart move blood clear obstructions (tumors, cholesterol, toxins, etc.).

Too many bitters cool, weaken, dry, constrict digestion, elimination, blood, etc. **Reduce** pungent, sour and salty tasting foods, herbs, which increase heat.

Anti-inflammatory drugs: Excess heat causes inflammation, burning. While thee are many good anti-inflammatory herbs (bitters), sometimes they are not strong enough, which is why Ibuprofen (800mg), etc. may be necessary. Check with your doctor.

Case history: near heart attack. I had changed my diet (lacto vegetarian) to include more cooked roots (rutabaga, turnips, beets) hot spices (black pepper, fresh ginger) and bitter herbs. I was also drinking a lot of coffee, which I rarely drank. I had been working at a soup kitchen at a local church two days a week where there is always coffee and cookies. I got into the habit. One day, a few months later I decided to have a couple of beers (alcohol is hot, dry). (1) That night I started experiencing the following symptoms: red face, increased heart rate (tachycardia), burning sensation, constriction in the chest, nausea, dizziness and fainting. I was overheated, dry and tight. I immediately adjusted my diet, added milk, increased raw vegetables, fruit, eliminated bitter herbs, coffee. It took four days before I returned to normal.

(2) A few days later my hair, became brittle, started breaking off in clumps and falling out. In two days, the hair was mostly gone, thinned out on the back of my head. Then the tops and the sides also thinned broke off. I researched hair loss and concluded that I was anemic, iron deficient, as iron deficiency (caused by low protein, lo aft diet, bitter herbs and sugar) will cause brittle hair and hair loss. I also consulted with a nurse (40 years experience). She checked me out, looked under my eyes, at my nails, etc. and said that I was iron deficient and that it would cause hair loss.

My diet was although lacto vegetarian, low protein, low fat (milk, cheese, beans, etc.) was not that low in iron as I was eating iron rich foods (dairy, beans, leafy greens, sesame seeds, etc.) but instead acidic (coffee and too much sugar), and bitter, which drained my blood, iron. My first instinct was to eat red meat, chicken, etc. (to rebuild quickly my blood, iron content), which I did for two days and right away my pulse rate started going up. I made a mistake, as protein and fat deficiency was not the cause, but instead coffee, sugar and bitter (drying, contracting) herbs. The answer was not more protein, fat but elimination of the offending habits, foods.

Many may wonder why **coffee**, 1- 2 cups per day for two to three months would have such a severe effect, when most, normal people who drink 3- 4 cups per day for twenty plus years do not have their hair fall out. The answer is these same people also eat red meat, chicken, turkey, eggs, etc. everyday, which somewhat offset the negative effects of coffee. For me, as a lacto vegetarian, the negative, deleterious effects of coffee were far more severe. This is a **cautionary tale to all vegetarians** (low resistance to bad, extreme foods).

Blood thinners I used to live in S. Florida (large elderly population). Many of my customers who were taking blood thinners long-term, complained about the increasing arthritis, melting, dissolving of bones in their hands and feet. Blood thinners thin the blood by removing excess protein, fat (cholesterol). **Protein and fat build thicken** the muscles, bones, organs, nerves, nails, etc. The best way to thin the blood is to stop thickening it via a reduction in animal protein, fat, fried foods, oil, while increasing fruits and vegetables. When you thin the blood, you thin, weaken all structure, function.

The heart and brain are largely a function of air (oxygen) and blood.

The lungs control respiration and are naturally moist (facilitates the exchange of gases (O_2 and CO_2). Too much water, mucous, phlegm reduces oxygen absorption, in the extreme, asphyxiating the brain. Weak digestion via cold, damp diets tend to cool and moisten the lungs, nose, sinuses and throat with excess mucous, phlegm.

The following are advanced symptoms of **cold phlegm (lungs) attacking the heart**

- Excess fluids can collect in the throat around the larynx (voice box) and cause a rattling sound. They can also leak dribble saliva out.

- Phlegm in the lungs decreases oxygen absorption, in the extreme, causing lethargic stupor, mental confusion, dullness, incoherence, muttering and a weak the tongue that hangs out. The heart opens up into the tongue (TCM).

Emotions also affect the heart, positively and negatively. Long-term sadness, depression and anger weaken the heart (stores the spirit). Unconditional love, forgiveness and even mindedness calm, relax and strengthen the heart. Avoid depressing and violent music, books, movies and people. Be happy.

"And thou shalt love the Lord, thy God with all thy heart, and with all thy soul, and with all thy mind, and with all thy strength: this is the first commandment. And the second is like, namely this, thou shalt love thy neighbor as thyself." Mark 12:30-31

"Blessed are the pure in heart for they shall see God" Mark 12:30

12

Lungs

The **lungs**, located in the chest, are composed of **five lobes** (rounded part of an organ separated from other parts of the organ by connective tissues): three in the right and two in the left. Lobes divide into **lobules** that connect to blood vessels, lymph. The lungs

- Control respiration
- Control skin, external immune system
- Assist the heart, circulation
- Assist large intestine (paired organ) defecation

Respiration controls the exchange of gases: oxygen (O_2) and carbon dioxide (CO_2) between the body and the environment. **Oxygen** purifies and nourishes the body. The brain uses 20% of the body's oxygen content. No cell, tissue can live without it for more than a few minutes. Carbon dioxide (poisonous waste: protein, fat and starch) increases respiration, heartbeat.

Green plants, trees, grasses (land and sea) via photosynthesis sunlight, take in, combine and transform carbon dioxide, water and minerals into oxygen and carbohydrates (fruit, vegetables, grains, beans, etc.).

Oxygen enters the body via the nose, throat → **lungs** → via the **bronchi** (two large lung channels) → **bronchioles** (smaller) → **alveoli** (air sacs, where gas exchange occurs) → **bloodstream** → **pulmonary vein** (carries oxygen-enriched blood from the lungs) → **heart**. The pulmonary artery carries CO_2 and old blood from the heart to the lungs for cleansing, oxygenation.

The lungs are naturally moist. Moisture, water facilitates the exchange of water-soluble gases: oxygen and carbon dioxide between the body and environment. Too much or too little decreases the oxygen exchange, weakens and distorts the breath.

- Coughing, mucous, phlegm, runny nose
- Reducing oxygen absorption, shortness of breath
- Coughing, hacking, snoring, sinusitis, sleep apnea
- Expectoration of mucous, phlegm, allergies

Normal body temperature (98.6°F), digestion, cooked foods, soups and spices heat, dry and thin bodily fluids. Colder, lower body temperatures thicken and slow fluids.

The spleen is the origin of damp and the **lungs its receptacle**. The lungs are located above the digestive organs (stomach, spleen, liver, small intestines, etc.). Three meals per day, spleen yang, fire (acid, enzymes) heat the digestive organs, which heat the rest of the body, especially the lungs. Heat rises.

Long-term **cold, damp**, low protein, low fat (soft dairy) and high carbohydrate (raw vegetables, fruits, juices, smoothies, sodas, cold drinks, ice water, sugar) diets cool, dampen, weaken, slow digestion and elimination, reduce nutrient absorption, blood, energy, body temperature, while increasing cold, damp.

Cold condenses. In nature, the colder temperatures of night and winter cool and harden water in the air or on the ground into the morning dew, rain, snow (white flakes) and or ice. Lower, colder body temperatures via long-term cold, damp diet, climate (winter, air conditioning) **thicken fluids** in the lungs, throat, sinuses, nose, breasts, vagina and uterus into excess mucous, phlegm, cysts, vaginal discharge and or yeast infection.

Excess fluids (water, mucous, phlegm) in the lungs, bronchi, alveoli, overtime

- Obstruct the nasal passages, bronchi, etc. restricting, distorting and or shortening the breath: breathlessness, snoring, asthma, sleep apnea, Chronic Obstructive Pulmonary Disease

- Decrease oxygen intake while increasing carbon dioxide in the blood, and the impulse to breathe, inhale, making it impossible to hold your breath.

- Obstruct the flow of blood and fluids causing dryness and inflammation in the sinuses (sinusitis), and bronchi (bronchitis). Smoking and bacterial infection can also be a cause.

- Cause splashing sounds in throat, chest

- Fosters **bacterial, fungal and viral growth**, which thrives in trapped, **stagnant fluids** (water, mucous, phlegm)

- Bronchitis, pleurisy, pneumonia

- Heats, dries, turns yellow or green clear, white mucous, phlegm that is harder, more difficult to dislodge forcing the lungs to violently cough, bark, hack to dislodge. A thick yellow coat indicates damp heat. Radishes, turnips and spices help dissolve mucous, phlegm.

Spices (cardamom, basil, ginger, cayenne, turmeric, etc.) used in cooking are heating, drying and toxic to many bacteria, viruses, fungi and mosquitoes via their essential oil content (hot, aromatic, purifying).

Bitter (cold) herbs are also antagonistic to many bacteria, viruses, fungi, etc. Too much bitter weakens digestion, constricts fluids, etc.

The lungs control the skin opening and closing of the pores, wei chi (external immune system) and body temperature

- **Closed pores** retain energy, heat while also acting as a shield in keeping out the six environmental evils (heat, cold, dryness, dampness, wind, and summer heat).

- **Open pores** help cool the body, eliminate excess energy, heat in the form of perspiration. via

Weak lungs via blood deficiency, sedentary lifestyle, obesity, smoking, etc. tend to keep the pores open allowing for external invasion, penetration of the six environmental evils, especially **cold, damp**.

Cold and damp air travels with the wind, and enters the upper part of the body: head, neck and shoulders, via open pores, just as air enters a house when the windows are open. Many mothers tell their children in winter to cover their necks and wear a hat before they go outside. They are not being fashionable, just smart.

An external, environmental attack of cold and damp (winter, air conditioning, living in a cold damp basement) tends to produce the following symptoms, associated with the **common cold**:   T

- Excess fluids, mucous and or phlegm in the lungs, throat, nose (stuffy) and sinuses

- Coughing, dry or wet cough (to dislodge mucous), shortness of breath, runny nose

- Dry, itchy, sore throat, headache, fever, sweating

- Stiff shoulders , aversion to cold

- Numbness and or shaking in the hands and feet

Most people catch cold because they are cold (weak). Human beings are naturally hot (normal body temperature 98.6°F). Any temperature, energy production below 98.6°F, in the extreme, tends to leave the body cold, weak, defenseless and vulnerable (open pores) to external attack, environmental extreme.

The body when cold, weak

- Drains, redirects blood from the extremities, head, arms and legs, into the chest and abdomen to protect vital organs. This leaves the extremities, **hands, feet and shoulders, cold, stiff.**

- Leaves its pores open, allow heat, energy and fluids (perspiration) to easily escape during the day causing **intermittent daytime sweating** (symptom of chi deficiency, lack of holding). The body is strongest (holding power) during the day.

- Raises its temperature, produces a **fever** to heat, dry excess cold, damp

- Causes aversion, fear of cold

- **Spices** reduce mucous, improve breathing

The **flu** is a more serious cold, with the following additional symptoms often lasting a week or more.

- Upper respiratory infection, nausea, vomiting
- Fatigue, malaise

Colds and flu's tend to occur during the winter, colder months. The majority of symptoms indicate deficiency, cold and damp.

Catching a cold is more prevalent in (1) **women, children and elderly** (tend to run cold) than in men (testosterone, high protein, fat diets), and (2) **Colder climates**, fall and winter than in spring and summer. Overexposure to air conditioning and or too many cold, damp foods, drinks tend to cause summertime colds. Additional symptoms; abdominal bloating, gas and loose stools generally indicate dietary cause.

The common cold in general is easy to cure if you can treat it at the onset (day 1 or 2) with its opposite: **excess heat** in the form of spicy vegetable soups, hot teas, hot baths, extra clothing, produce fever, perspiration. Decrease all cold foods, drinks, milk, ice cream, sugar, sodas, ice water, etc. **Keeping the body hot** is the key to a strong immunity.

The hotter middle diet, **spices**, (cardamom, basil, cayenne, black pepper, turmeric, ginger, etc.) is recommended. The spicy (pungent) taste stimulates the lungs helps disperse, dry fluids. Too many spices dry the lungs. Herbal remedies (golden seal and echinacea) also help.

Mushrooms, black fungus, poria (fungus) and spices drain excess mucous, phlegm. Check with your doctor first. Many Asian women regularly eat fungus

Case history: I was visiting a friend and his wife in Fort Meyers, Fl. where his parents lived. They had flown in from Seattle where they live. When I got there, he was coughing up a storm, non-stop. He said it was his allergies.

I said it was a **cold** (coughing, runny nose, stiff shoulders). I told him he needed to eat hot foods at which time he held up his beer. Alcohol is hot, dry, which made his cough, drier, worse. I went into his mother's kitchen and made him a hot, spicy vegetable soup. I threw in every hot spice that I could find. He gobbled the soup down (two bowls) and within 20 minutes, his cough and runny nose ceased. Before the soup, he had been coughing every ten minutes.

Excess heat via environment (hot, dry climate), **diet** (alcohol, coffee and smoking) and blood deficiency (blood is moistening) **heats and dries** the body, lungs:

- Wind heat (summer cold)
- High fever
- Thirst, cough, dryness
- Sore throat (swollen red)
- Runny nose with yellow mucous
- Tongue red on the sides with or without a yellow coating. The absence of a thick or thin yellow coating indicates the cause to be external (climate), acute and not internal, dietary.

Severe childhood trauma, sadness, depression, grief, excessive sitting, sedentary lifestyle, excessive sex and chronic illnesses drain, weaken the lungs.

Honey, sugar, milk, raw beets and white fungus (contraindicated yeast infections) help moisten the lungs as do lesser hot spices, smoking. Peppermint tea helps counter the drying effects of smoking.

Regular, daily exercise, walking 30 minutes twice a day and deep abdominal breathing (pages 297- 300) strengthens the lungs, increases respiration, circulation, immunity; elimination, etc. help dissolve lung tumors.

Smoking is very damaging to the lungs, kidneys, heart, etc. The lungs will recover; self-clean when given the chance, correct nutrition. Read the following story.

Case history (smoker): One of my long-term customers was an eighty-year-old man, John who always bought the same supplements, selenium and lecithin. I asked him why. He told me, a little irritated, that he had just gotten back from Hollywood Presbyterian Hospital for his biannual check up with his pulmonary doctor.

They took x-rays and the first doctor exclaimed that John had probably never smoked a cigarette in his life. John laughed and told the doctor he was a heavy-duty smoker, two packs per day for 40 years but had quit for the last 20 years. The doctor did not believe him. He said he was going to call the head of the pulmonary department to examine the x-rays. An older man came in, said he could spot a casual smoker by his x-rays, examined the pictures and said beyond a doubt that John had never smoked in his life. John was lying. He was buying selenium and lecithin because his doctor 20 years ago told him that if he did not give up smoking and alcohol that he was going get cancer and heart disease. John refused saying he liked smoking and dinking. The doctor said fine and advised selenium for lungs and lecithin for heart. **Mullein** also helps dispel lung heat and congestion. **Raw red beets**, juice supposed helps dissolve lung tumors

Excessive sex, cold drinks, overwork, etc. also weaken the kidneys, kidney yang, which weakens, shortens the inhalation. Kidney yang supports lung yang, anchors the breath.

13

Kidneys

The kidneys (bean shaped paired organs) are located on the rear wall of the abdomen in the small of the lower back on either side of the spine and connect via ureters to the urinary bladder. The kidneys have several functions.

1. Store and transform jing sexual essence (TCM)

2. Rule the bones, marrow, sex organs, etc. (TCM)

3. Filter the blood, remove and combine nitrogenous wastes (from protein and fat digestion), urea, and water into urine that passes down into the urinary bladder for temporary storage, eventual excretion

4. Regulate electrolytes (positive and negative ions). Electrolytes conduct electrical current, which regulates all function.

5. Regulate pH (acid and alkaline balance), which helps buffer (stabilizes hydrogen ion concentration) and cleanse the blood. The pH scale ranges from 1 – 14. A pH of seven is neutral. Below seven is acid, above, alkaline. Normal body, blood pH is approximately **7.35- 7.45**. Any number above (alkalosis) or below (acidosis), in the extreme, sickens the body. Protein, fat and starch (grain, starchy vegetables) are acidic. Raw fruits, vegetables and spices are alkaline.

6. Control urinary bladder, urination

Jing is the fundamental, material substance of life governing birth, growth and development. It is stored in the left kidney as kidney yin and transformed by the right kidney (kidney yang, gate of fire) into

- Marrow, bones, brain, spinal chord
- Sex organs, head hair, teeth
- Original chi is the initial stimulus of all function.

The amount of jing is fixed at birth. Its decline (starts after sexual maturity) signals the end of youth, and beginning of middle and old age.

Blood, protein and fat builds and fuels all structure function, including jing.

- **Too little protein, fat**, in the extreme, decreases thin the blood, which in turn, consumes jing as a replacement fuel.

- **Too much animal protein, fat, fried foods, *caffeine, alcohol, smoking and stimulant drugs** overheats the body stimulates sexual desire accelerates the consumption of jing. Many religions advise the vegetarian diet and avoidance of alcohol, drugs, etc. to reduce sexual desire, body consciousness. *Cardamom helps detox caffeine.

Excessive sex, masturbation, sex accelerates the consumption, burning of jing, **aging, weakening** the kidneys, bones, marrow, brain, hair, etc. Sex is especially weakening for man as orgasm, ejaculation causes a great loss of energy (jing is high protein, high fat) and unconsciousness. Eastern religions advise all men to withhold, **forgo the ejaculation, orgasm**, when having recreational sex. Orgasm is less damaging to women (menstruation).

Forgoing the orgasm not only conserves jing but also extends lovemaking. Give up the small (orgasm) for the greater (longer lovemaking, healthier life). Jing is the fountain of youth when full, and the harbinger of old age, disease when less, declining.

Sex also stimulates, increases body consciousness. Many spiritual disciplines advocate **celibacy** to redirect jing (water) up the spine into the higher chakras, spiritual centers (fire) to increase spiritual consciousness, instead of moving down into the lower chakras (digestion, elimination and sex), which increases material consciousness and unhappiness.

Kidney pathologies are defined in terms of yin and yang. Kidney yin (jing) builds fuels and moistens all structure (yin), function (yang), including kidney yang. Kidney yin is never in excess, only decline. Kidney yin deficiency (stage 6) drains, thins all yin (moisture, substance) and yang. Old age, poor diet, caffeine, alcohol, drugs, smoking, blood deficiency, excessive sex, chronic illness, bulimia, overwork, heredity and or living in an excessively hot, dry climate drains kidney yin, yang.

Kidney yin deficiency (long-term)

- Dry mouth and throat, night sweats, and or malar flush (partial facial flushing) are caused by lack, deficiency of Kidney yin, blood, which dries, heats the body, especially during the night when body, circulation, blood is less active, moistening. Total flushing (entire face, body), is caused by excess heat too, much building, protein, fat.

- Thins, dries the skin, hair, eyes, secretions, etc.

- Thins, dries and weakens the bones, teeth

- Dries, heats the body, brain during the night, which stimulates the brain, thinking, dreaming, restlessness, insomnia.

- Thins, dries and weakens the marrow, brain, causing poor concentration, memory loss, dizziness, vertigo and or loss of consciousness.

- Causes "soft" ringing in the ears (tinnitus), as opposed to loud (excess, liver heat). The kidneys open up into the ears.

- Weakens kidney yang

Kidney yang stimulates all function (yang): digestion (spleen yang), respiration (lung yang, page 138), circulation (heart yang) and reproduction (kidney yang).

Kidney yin (jing) and blood deficiency, old age, sex, orgasm, alcohol, caffeine, drugs and extreme cold via climate and diet (excessive milk, ice cream, tropical fruits, fruit juices, cold drinks and bitter herbs) weaken kidney yang.

Kidney yang deficiency (long-term)

- Causes fear (cardinal symptom)

- Cause coldness (Kidney yang warms the body)

- Weakens, pains the lower back and legs, especially the knees (cardinal symptoms). The kidneys (located in lower back) rule the bones.

- Weakens digestion, spleen yang, causes loose stools at daybreak and or organ prolapse (uterus, rectum, etc.). Spleen yang uplifts, holds the organs in their places.

- Increases and thickens water increasing the frequency, urge and flow of urination. It also causes water to overflow into the legs and ankles (edema). Kidney yang controls water metabolism, heats the bladder, thins the urine.

- Weakens the bladder causes leaking during the night (nocturnal emissions)

- Long-term blood, protein and fat deficiency also weakens spleen yang, holding, causing sinking, prolapse. Energy (chi, yang) and blood (protein, fat) hold the skin, organs, bones, thoughts, etc. in their place.

- Weakens the lungs, heart decreases the breath, inhalation, circulation, blood flow to the head, face: bright, white complexion (cold). Blood is red. Kidney yang anchors the breath, inhalation.

- Causes premature ejaculation (lack of holding), impotence and infertility in women. Kidney yang heats the body, sexual organs, transforms jing into ovum, move the egg through the ovaries and fallopian tubes down into the uterus.

- Cools, moistens and thickens fluids in the uterus, vagina into clear or white mucous discharges, and or yeast infection.

- Burns less fluid moves less blood (red) causing the tongue to become pale, swollen and wet.

The kidneys, jing are nourished by protein, fat (especially red meat), **black** foods (black beans, black fungus, black sesame seeds, black dates, rhemannia, etc.), warmth, sexual moderation and the salty taste. Salt helps move water.

Too much salt (includes sea salt) tightens and weakens the kidneys increasing water retention (edema). Excess cold via diet (cold drinks, ice water, bitter herbs, ice cream, etc.) and climate (winter, A/C, lying or cold ground, sleeping in a cold damp basement) also weakens (cools) the kidneys, drains kidney yang. Cover and wrap the lower back with extra clothing to protect against cold and wind, drafts.

Remedies are important when curing disease as is removal of the cause. Non-removal weakens all remedies, while also prolonging disease.

14

Asian Diagnosis and Treatment

Structure→ function→ **symptom**→ health, disease

Diagnosis identifies disease (abnormal function) via examination of symptoms produced by one or more of the bodily structures (glands, organs, bones, blood, etc.). Every structure function does nothing more than build up (thicken, heat, expand, etc.) and break down (thin, cool, contract, etc.) largely via diet. The correct balance, amounts of building up and breaking down produces health via the correct, normal amount of structure function. The incorrect, too much or too little building or cleansing, in the extreme, produces disease via too much or too little structure function.

Food→ digestion→ **blood** → structure→ function→

Asian diagnosis defines every structure, function (healthy, diseased), nutrient, food, herb, climate, etc. in terms of energy, as all matter is a reflection, form of energy. Energy is always moving, changing, **building up** (yang, hot) **and breaking down** (yin, cold), which in turn, builds up (thickens, heats, dries, tightens, etc.), and breaks down (thins, cools, moistens, loosens, etc.) its material form (gas, solid, liquid).

Controlling energetic opposites (hot and cold) largely via diet (building and cleansing foods, herbs), is the key to controlling the body, health and disease.

I. Building nutrients, foods
- Protein and fat (saturated and unsaturated fat)
- (1) Red meat (2) Chicken (3) turkey (4) Fish
- (5) Eggs (6) Hard cheese (7) Soft dairy
- (8) Beans, nuts, seeds

Building nutrients, foods build, thicken fuel, heat, dry, moisten and tighten.

Too much protein, fat symptoms, diseases
- Blood clots, high cholesterol, tumors, cancer
- Plaque, atherosclerosis high blood pressure
- Congested, swollen liver high uric acid, gout
- Sexual organs dysmenorrhea, prostatitis
- Skin dry, scaly, oily, acne, warts, boils, psoriasis
- Obesity, insomnia, higher body temperature
- **Treatment** colder middle diet, meal plan

Too little protein, fat cold symptoms, diseases
- Thin blood, anemia, low cholesterol, fatigue
- Poor circulation, coldness,
- Thin, racked hair, skin and nails, eczema bleeding
- Amenorrhea, infertility, miscarriage, impotence
- Autoimmune illnesses
- **Treatment** hotter middle diet, meal plan

II. Cleansing nutrients, foods
- Water, minerals, vitamins, enzymes
- (1) Salt, minerals (2) Bitter herbs (3) Sugar
- (4) Water (5) Fruit (6) Vegetables (7) Grain

Cleansing nutrients, foods cool, cleanse, moisten, soften, loosen, reduce, thin, slow, contract, sink, relax and calm. Too many fruits, vegetables, juices, cold drinks, etc. dilute, weaken and slow digestion and elimination, reduce nutrient absorption, blood, energy.

Too much cleansing cold, damp symptoms
- Stomach: gas, bloating
- U. bladder: profuse urination, bladder infection
- Large intestine: loose stools, constipation
- **Treatment** hotter middle diet, meal plan

Too little cleansing dry, hot symptoms
- Stomach: heartburn, reflux
- Urinary: bladder scanty urination
- Large intestine: dry stools, constipation
- **Treatment** colder middle diet, meal plan

Building and cleansing nutrients, foods, herbs, etc. can easily be adjusted, increased or decreased to build up or break down structure, function that is too thick, thin, hard, soft, fast, slow, hot, cold, dry, damp, etc.

Hot (building, yang) and cold (cleansing, yin) is a simple, **general diagnosis and treatment plan** that requires complete knowledge of biology, as every structure function, not only works together, but many times share similar symptoms, diseases but not necessarily causes or treatments.

The **common cold** is a good example. It has the following symptoms:
- Mucous, coughing, shortness of breath
- Cold hands, feet, stiff shoulders and fever

Structure→ function→ symptoms→

- The lungs control respiration, breathing
- The spleen controls digestion, blood and dampness
- The heart controls blood, circulation

Mucous, coughing and shortness of breath identify the lungs and or spleen. Cold hands, feet and stiff shoulders identify the heart, lungs and or spleen

The lungs are naturally moist. Moisture facilitates the exchange of gases (oxygen, carbon dioxide).

Too much moisture (mucous, phlegm) clogs, weakens the lungs, respiration:

- Coughing, shortness of breath, sore throat

Colder body temperatures via cold, damp environment (winter, air conditioning) or diet (milk, soft cheese, ice cream, salads, fruits, juices, cold drinks) cool, slow and harden fluids in the lungs, throat, sinuses, etc. into excess mucous, phlegm.

The spleen controls digestion. Digestion transforms food into blood. It also heats and dries (thins fluids) the body, especially the lungs, which are located above the digestive organs. Digestive fire, heat (three meals a day) naturally rises up into the lungs, throat, mouth, etc. heating and drying.

Protein and fat fuel digestion. Too little protein, fat or too many cold damp foods: drinks, in the extreme, cool, weaken, decrease digestion, nutrient absorption, blood, energy. Chronically weak digestion and or blood deficiency lowers body temperature, which cools and hardens fluids in the lungs, sinuses, etc. into

- Mucous, phlegm, the same way, colder temperatures cool harden water in the air, into the morning dew, rain, snow and ice.

The heart controls circulation, blood. Chronically thin (deficient) blood decreases circulation, especially to the extremities: head, arms and legs causing

- Cold hands, cold feet, shaking, stiff shoulders

Long-term cold, damp, low protein, low fat diets, chronic illness and cold, damp climates tend to cause symptoms associated with the common cold.

The common cold caused by environmental cold is generally easy, can quickly be cured if treated at the onset, day one or two with hot, spicy soups, hot baths, alcohol (in tea), sweating, additional clothing, etc.

Symptoms of the common cold caused by chronic, long-term cold, damp diet, blood (protein, fat) deficiency require longer, stronger (hotter) treatment time (months) to recuperate, rebuild the body, blood.

Most disease travels through the body just as food, nutrients travel through the stomach, small intestine into the blood, arteries, heart, bones, brain, skin, hair, etc. The following are the general stages of dietary disease. Poor diet causes most disease.

- **Stage 1** Cause: Poor diet weakens
- **Stage 2** Digestion: abdominal bloating, gas, pain
- **Stage 3** Elimination: loose stools, constipation
- **Stage 4** Blood: fatigue, pallor, tension, coldness
- **Stage 5** Circulation: numbness, inflammation, pain, shaking, arthritis, etc.
- **Stage 6** Organ dysfunction: diabetes, psoriasis, autoimmune illnesses, heart attack, cancer

Disease can occur quickly or take longer (months, years) to develop. **Acute** diseases (common cold, sore throat, etc.) occur quickly, and in general, can cure quickly if treated at the onset, beginning, day one or two, via proper diet and herbs. **Chronic** diseases take months, years to develop and consequently months, years to heal, cure, depending on severity.

There are no quick, fast cures, only positive attitude, patience, discipline, etc. when treating chronic disease.

It never hurts, and many times is wise to see a doctor, get x-rays, blood work, etc. Regardless of cause and cure, you still have to eat well. The body, healthy and diseased determines diet, choice of food. Health widens the diet, disease narrows.

There are many ways to diagnose. **Energetic diagnosis**: hot (building, yang) and cold (cleansing, yin) is the easiest diagnosis, as everything (biology, diet, etc.) has an overall hot or cold nature.

Simple hot and cold diagnosis, exercise: Get a blank piece of paper and fold it in half. **On one side, write hot, building, and on the other, cold, cleansing.** List your diet, foods, herbs, age, gender, climate, symptoms, diseases (Section II), accordingly.

HOT (pitta)	**COLD** (kapha, vata)
Red meat, chicken, eggs turkey, hard cheese, root vegetables, alcohol, hot spices, coffee, smoking spring, summer, male, tumors, cancer, obesity	Soft dairy, sugar, fruit, juice, raw vegetables, water, cold drinks, bitter herbs, fall, winter, female, anemia, fatigue, thin, amenorrhea, autoimmune

Examine the list and identify the imbalance. **One side will always be greater**. If you cannot decide which one is greater, ask yourself or others if you are too hot (aggressive, anxious, too much energy, etc.) or too cold (passive, laid back, tired, etc.), and then re-examine your diet, surroundings, symptoms, etc. They (input, cause and output, effect) should match. **Cold** diets, herbs, environments cause cold symptoms, diseases. **Hot** causes hot. **Deficiency** causes deficiency. **Excess** causes excess. **Dry** causes dry. **Damp** causes damp.

This is your energetic profile. If you feel, look and act well, your balance is correct, healthy. If not, your balance is too extreme: too hot or too cold.

The solution, treatment plan for all dietary diseases is simple: **(1) Colder middle diet** for hot, high protein, high fat diseases **(2) Hotter middle diet** for cold, low protein, low fat diseases. The right choice makes you feel better, the wrong choice, worse.

Hot and cold is a simple diagnosis and treatment plan. It is also limited, less defined. Biological, structural and functional identification, is more detailed, informative, as every structure, function, healthy and diseased is nutrient, food, herb, climate, symptom, etc. specific. The following tables list common symptoms, diseases according to chi, blood, jing, body fluids and organ function. Many symptoms can have hot and cold causes.

I. Chi, blood, fluids, jing and wind

A. Chi

Deficiency (cold, vata)
- Fatigue, perspires easily, sleeps a lot, feels cold
- Breathlessness, hard to project voice
- Drops things easily, lack of appetite, pale tongue

Stagnation (hot or cold)
- Mental depression, mood swings, hot flash
- Frequent sighing, tongue is dark or purplish
- Distention in chest, ribs, abdominal distention
- Muscle tension, pain, soreness, varies in location

Sinking (cold)
- Bearing down sensation, fatigue, weariness
- Depression, bruises easily, varicose veins
- Sagging skin, prolapse (stomach, uterus)

Rebellious (hot or cold)
- Belching, nausea, vomiting, hiccoughs
- Heartburn, headaches, restlessness, hot flash

B. Blood

Deficiency (cold, vata)
- Pal face, mouth and tongue, pain, inflammation
- Dry lips, eyes and skin, numbness, poor vision
- Shaking, forgetfulness, dizziness, weakness
- Amenorrhea, infertility, miscarriage, insomnia

Stagnation (hot, pitta)
- Dark complexion, purple lips and nails
- Swelling of organs, abdominal masses, arthritis
- Tumors, cancer, fixed, stabbing pain, tension
- Dysmenorrhea, menstrual clots, PMS
- High blood pressure, stroke

Heat (hot, pitta)
- Bleeding, blood in the stools, urine
- Acne, boils, psoriasis, itching, scratching
- Dysmenorrhea, insomnia, red tongue

C. Fluids

Deficiency→ vata
- Dry skin, mouth, lips, tongue, nose, sexual fluids
- Dry stools, scanty urination, hoarse voice

Excess→ kapha
- Mucous, phlegm, snoring, sleep apnea
- Loose stools, cysts, cellulite, sweet body odor

Phlegm→ kapha
- Phlegm nodules in thyroid gland, lymph gland
- Bone deformities, arthritis
- Cysts, stones, fibrocystic breast

D. Jing

- Premature aging, graying and loss of hair, fear
- Bone, tooth loss, hair loss, impotence, infertility

E. Wind → vata (air)

- Spasms, tremors, paralysis, stiffness, numbness
- Dizziness, vertigo, convulsions, seizure, stroke

II Organ Function

A. Digestion

Spleen
- Abdominal bloating, loose stools, diarrhea
- Blood deficiency, fatigue, worry
- Feeling heavy, organ prolapse

Stomach
- Nausea, vomiting, acid reflux, sour breath
- Stomach pain, GIRD, GERD

Small Intestine
- Abdominal pain, borborygmus tongue ulcers
- Bearing down sensation (abdomen)

B. Elimination

Urinary Bladder
- Kidney, bladder stones, gravel, sand in urine
- Frequent, pale, cloudy, burning urination
- Urinary tract infection, incontinence

Large intestine
- Diverticulitis (pockets), dry stools
- Constipation, pain in rectum, hemorrhoids

C. Blood cleansing, digestion

Liver
- Inability to digest fat, poor nail growth
- Migraines, pain in abdomen (right flank)
- Anger, irritability, poor vision (floaters)
- Red eyes, loud ringing in ears (tinnitus)
- Shoulder, neck tension Insomnia (11 P. M. - 3 A.M.)
- Acne, psoriasis, warts, tumors, high cholesterol

Gall bladder
- Nausea, vomiting bitter fluids, bitter taste
- Gall stones, jaundice, right side piercing pain

D. Respiration

Lungs
- Mucous, phlegm, cough, shortness of breath
- Asthma, bronchitis, pleurisy, pneumonia
- Sleep apnea, fullness, pain in the chest
- Easily catches colds, grief, sadness

E. Circulation
Heart
- Palpitations, chest, arm pain (left side)
- Insomnia, excessive dreaming, poor memory
- Restlessness, anxiety, tongue ulcers, sores
- Atherosclerosis

F. Reproduction

Kidneys
- Hair and bone loss, weak, lower back, knees
- Fall, break bones easily, incontinence, insomnia
- Kidney stones, nocturnal emissions, night sweats
- No sex drive, infertility, poor memory

Kidneys
- Dry mouth, throat at night, edema in the ankles
- Cold body, limbs, pale, white complexion, fear

Tongue diagnosis: The fluids of the stomach normally overflow onto the tongue creating a thin white coating. Too many cold foods and drinks tend to create excess fluids in the stomach that overflow onto the tongue creating a thick white coating. Too many hot foods, alcohol, etc. tends to cause a thick yellow coating. Yellow and green are the colors of heat. White and clear are the colors of cold. A thick tongue coating indicates dampness while thin or no coating indicates yin (fluid, blood, jing) deficiency. For more information: **Tongue Diagnosis in Chinese Medicine** by Giovanni Maciocia

There is also **constitutional and conditional medicine,** diagnosis and treatment. Everyone is born with a certain constitution: male, female, yin, yang, vata, pitta, kapha, blood type (page 175), etc. While constitutions do not change, conditions (internal and external) do. Men tend to be hot and therefore need to eat more fruits, vegetables and bitter herbs and less animal, hot spices, alcohol, coffee, etc. However, a man's condition can become too cold via climate (cold) or diet (cold, damp, low protein, low fat); therefore, he will need to eat more animal, cooked foods, spices and less soft dairy, raw, cold, etc. The same

There are many ways to self diagnose. A medical dictionary is necessary, as is a medical consultation, blood work, etc. I highly recommend

Dictionary of Medical Terms
Mikel A. Rothenberg, M.D. & Charles F. Chapman
Barron's Educational Series, Inc. (c) 2000
Paperback: 500 pages $6.95 (2002)

Treatment for dietary disease is always the same: middle diet, meal plan (pages 54- 58), adjusted accordingly. Herbs (includes spices) are often advised. Herbs, in general are more powerful, healing in the short-run but tend to be harmful in the long. **Some herbs may conflict with prescription medications.** Check with your doctor.

Every food, herb, nutrient, etc is structure function specific, health and disease. Research every herb in order to get a more complete understanding. The following is a list of authors and their books that I regularly use. It was in **Energetics of Western Herbs, Volumes I; II** by Peter Holmes that I discovered that peppermint oil was a cure for toothache, infected nerves (pages 281-3). I highly recommend:

- **Yoga of Herbs** Dr. David Frawley, Dr. Vasant Lad
- **Ayurvedic Healing** Dr. David Frawley, O.M.D.
- **Energetics of Western Herbs, I, II** by Peter Holmes
- **Chinese Herbs with Common Foods** Henry C. Lu
- **Diet and Salad** by N.W. Walker
- **Chinese Health Care Secrets** by Henry B. Lin
- **Healing with Whole Foods** by Paul Pitchford
- **Asian Health Secrets** by Letha Hadady, D. Ac.
- **The Tao of Nutrition** by Maoshing Ni, Ph.D. C.A.
- **The Tao of Healthy Eating** by Bob Flaws, prolific author, Blue Poppy Press, best TCM books
- **Prescription for Nutritional Healing** by Phyllis A. Balch, CNC and James P. Balch, M.D.

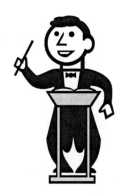

Section III. Pathology

Important information

This section is limited to the Eastern view that lifestyle: poor diet, excessive sex and lack of exercise tend to cause most disease, and do not preclude medical consultation and or treatment. Please consult with a physician before making any changes to your diet, exercise program, etc.

All disease is defined by its symptoms not by its names. There will always be major and minor, initial and latter symptoms. It is the initial major symptoms and their associated structure functions that must cure, to cure all subsequent symptoms, diseased (abnormal) structure functions. Know the whole before diagnosing and treating any one part.

There will always be stories of miraculous healing via "miracle" foods, herbs, etc. which generally does not occur without other miracles, long-term comprehensive changes in diet, lifestyle. Miracles are generally the tip of the iceberg.

15

"A" Diseases

ACNE

Acne is an **inflammatory (hot)** disease of the sebaceous glands primarily affecting the face, shoulders and back producing raised, red lesions, pustules, blackheads, etc. Protein and fat build, fuel all structure function, including the skin. Too much protein, fat, especially animal, fried foods, oil and sugar (excess sugar turns into fat) thicken and heat the blood. Thick blood, in the extreme, thickens, heats, reddens the skin, face, shoulders and back producing raised, red, hard painful, oily pimples; pus, boils, bumps, warts, moles, psoriasis, tumors or dry flaky skin. Heat rises pushes fat up and out. For "hot" acne, psoriasis, etc. the colder middle diet, burdock tea is recommended. Hormones can also be a cause. For more info: Skin Diseases (page 276)

AIDS, HIV

AIDS (Acquired Immune **Deficiency** Syndrome) is acquired developed and or contracted via sex, drugs, unsanitary needles, blood transfusions or long-term poor diet. It tends to affect men (jing depletion) more than women and is often associated with the HIV immunodeficiency virus, which can invade and weaken the immune system, white blood cells, T lymphocytes, leading to total breakdown, infection and or cancer. HIV does not always develop into AIDS (rate is 20- 50%). AIDS, HIV are cold, deficient stage 6 diseases.

All disease including HIV, AIDS require food for growth. Long-term cold, damp, low protein, low fat, high sugar, juices, cold drinks, caffeine and drugs weaken, slow (2) digestion, (3) elimination, (4) blood, (5) circulation and (6) immunity.

Excessive sex, masturbation, orgasm in men is a major contributing factor. Jing (sexual essence) is the fundamental, material substance of life, fountain of youth (vitality, full, lush hair, firm, glowing skin, strong bones, etc.) when full and the specter of old age, when low. Excessive sex (daily), alcohol, caffeine (very weakening), drugs and smoking accelerate the consumption, burning of jing, aging drying and weakening the body: digestion, immunity, etc.

The more a man ejaculates orgasms, the faster he physically and mentally ages, deteriorates. TCM advises all men to reduce sex, avoid ejaculation, especially as one gets older. Celibacy enables one to retain their essence, use it for higher purposes.

Homosexual men who have excessive sex, masturbation, orgasm (daily +), take drugs and eat a long-term low protein, low fat and sweet diet (fruits, juices, sugar, alcohol, etc.) and or intravenous drugs users (sharing needles) tend to contract or develop HIV, AIDS faster than any other group. The incidence of AIDS is very low among lesbians and heterosexuals.

HIV and AIDS are more common in countries where there is mass starvation, poor hygiene or exposure to raw sewage. The AIDS virus can stay alive outside the body 10- 11 days if kept in sewage (broken down, deteriorated food, waste product).

Not everyone exposed to HIV, AIDS, develops HIV or AIDS. It depends on the immune system, overall health. HIV, depending on severity is curable, AIDS more difficult to cure. The middle diet adjusted accordingly, is recommended, in addition to no, or sexual moderation.

Stages of AIDS/ HIV
1. Long-term cold, damp low protein, low fat, high carbohydrate diet, excessive sex
2. Indigestion, abdominal bloating, gas
3. Diarrhea, constipation, gas, pain
4. Anemia, fatigue, pallor, weight loss
5. Poor circulation pain, inflammation, numbness, skin rashes, dull headaches, etc.
6. Mouth lesions, sores, thrush, swollen gums, glands, coughing, sore throat, shortness of breath, pain in the joints and muscles
7. Prolonged, unexplained fatigue, lasting fever, speech impairment, memory loss, lesions, Pneumonia, Candidal Esophagitis, Primary lymphoma, Kaposi' sarcoma (tumor), herpes

Aging

Aging is a function of fuel and time (use). The more fuel (jing, protein and fat) the body burns the faster it ages (dries, weakens). Old age is also a cause.

Jing (sexual essence, protein and fat rich) is the primary substance, fuel, fountain of youth. It is limited at birth. You get one fuel tank. At its peak (men: late teens, women: late twenties), jing produces thick, colorful hair, strong skin, bones, muscles, energy, memory, healing ability, etc. In its decline, the body ages, dries, weakens, etc. Sex, masturbation, orgasm, consumes, burns the most, which is why sex is reduced as one ages.

Less sex or celibacy is highly beneficial to physical, mental and spiritual well-being, especially for men, who experience the greater loss, often lose consciousness after orgasm. Seeds (pumpkin, sesame, sunflower, etc.) nourish jing.

Coffee, caffeine excessively drains, burns jing

Too much protein, fat especially animal accelerates the consumption, burning of jing as does stress, lack of sleep, overwork, alcohol, coffee, drugs and smoking. Too little protein, fat, also consumes jing, as it is used as a replacement fuel for dietary protein, fat, especially when working hard or having sex.

Eating less extends life. "To lengthen thy life, lessen thy meals." The colder middle diet, spiritual practices: meditation, kindness, generosity, unconditional love, vegetarian diet and deep abdominal breathing (page 297) extend youthful appearance, life.

Alzheimer's disease

Alzheimer's is a common type of dementia that generally affects men and women, in their later years. Dementia is a progressive state of mental decline, physical deterioration of the nerves, producing the following symptoms: short-term memory loss, confusion, disorientation, violence and or stupor. It is generally a cold, deficient disease. When autopsied, the brains, including cerebral arteries of Alzheimer's patients tended to be **dry, brown and shrunken** (deficient blood). The brain (one-third blood vessels) is normally red (blood, arteries) in color. Dry, brown suggest a lack of blood flow due to deficient blood and or clogged arteries.

Long-term blood, protein and fat deficiency via long-term low protein, low fat diets tend to starve, weaken, dry and shrink the nerves, brain, causing decreased mental function, memory lapse and in the extreme, dementia. Mercury, aluminum poisoning, excessive sex, caffeine, alcohol and smoking can also be a cause. The middle diet, meal plan adjusted accordingly is recommended regardless of the extreme. Reduce, avoid, coffee, caffeine, alcohol, smoking and sex.

Anal Fissure

Case History: A friend of mine developed an anal fissure (tear in the intestines). He went to his doctor who told him that there was no cure. The best that he could do was operate, sew it back together; however the operation, procedure might make him temporarily incontinent (urine, bowels) and or impotent. I told him to skip the operation and eat the colder middle diet: while eliminating fried foods, bran (coarse), etc. His fissure healed. His original diet was high protein, fat, starch and low vegetables, fruit.

Anemia

Anemia (blood *deficiency* in TCM) is a reduction in the number of red blood cells and or amount of hemoglobin. Red blood cells carry oxygen, nutrients and waste products to and from every cell. The following are symptoms of anemia: fatigue, coldness in the extremities, facial pallor, pale lips and nails, loss of appetite, amenorrhea (little or no period), arthritis, difficulty concentrating, headaches and or constipation.

Protein and fat (high in iron) build, thicken, fuel and heat the blood and all structure, function.

Too little thins, weakens and cools. Low protein, low fat diets, in the extreme, reduce, thin the blood. Iron supplements (constipating) do little to correct blood deficiency unlike red meat, chicken, hard cheese, brewers yeast, etc. Too many raw fruits, vegetables, juices and cold drinks weaken and dilute digestion, acid, enzymes, reducing nutrient absorption, thinning the blood.

Anemia, blood deficiency (thin blood) tends to attack women more so than men. Many women tend to eat low protein, low fat (milk, yogurt, soft cheese, beans, etc.) and high carbohydrate diets. They also menstruate lose blood, three to seven days every month for thirty plus years, both of which contribute to anemia, blood deficiency.

Children tend to develop anemia due to age (under-developed, weak digestion, assimilation) and diet. Western children tend to eat poorly: too much milk, cereal, sugar, juice, soda, cold drinks, etc. Chronic illness, radiation, drugs and surgery can also cause anemia. The hotter middle diet, raw beets is recommended for dietary anemia. Pernicious anemia is more serious, caused by a lack of Vitamin B12 (found primarily in animal foods).

Anger

Anger is frustrated desire, the inability to accept and work with things as they are, instead trying to force loud, quick and ineffective resolutions via critique, condescension, violence, etc. It can have mental (fear, lack of faith) and physical causes neither of which is an excuse to act poorly, as all emotions are choices Anger that causes negation of bad habits is positive.

.

On a physical level, excess energy, protein, fat, trapped in the blood (clots, cholesterol), arteries (plaque, atherosclerosis, high blood pressure); liver, muscles (tension), etc. can frustrate, overheat the mind, giving it an excuse to release its trapped energy violently. Anger, like all emotions, despite the circumstances, is a choice.

In TCM, the liver is the organ associated with anger. It stores, cleanses and releases the blood. Too much protein, fat (especially animal), in the extreme, tends to clog, harden and weaken the liver. Less cholesterol, fat are removed, more stays in the blood (high cholesterol) and arteries (plaque, atherosclerosis, high blood pressure). Overtime, the body becomes clogged, hard, inflexible overheated, pressurized which can frustrate, anger the mind, causing it to seek a quick, violent release of trapped energy.

The colder middle diet, vegetarian, more raw fruits and vegetables, bitter herbs (page 54), no alcohol, dugs, more exercise (dissipates excess energy) spiritual practices, love, forgiveness, meditation, fasting and moderate lifestyle helps eliminate anger.

Anxiety

Anxiety is a state of mild to severe apprehension that may causes rapid heartbeat, perspiration, panic attacks, etc. **Case history:** One of my customers (60 years old, vegetarian, S. Florida) was having frequent anxiety attacks. When I counseled her, she was screaming, yelling from one anxiety attack to another. To calm and control her outbursts, I taught her how to breathe deeply, abdominally. My initial impression was excess heat, as her energy was all over the place. She seemed extremely hot, out of control (lack of holding).

I discovered (via consultation form) that she had uncontrollable urination: kidney yang deficiency (outweighs all other symptoms). Her condition was one of extreme deficiency caused by long-term low protein, low fat vegetarian diet. Deficiency (inability to control) not excess, caused her anxiety. Her diet was anemic: too little building, blood to strengthen, control, moisten her energy fire, so she became hot, dry, irritable, etc.

I recommended the hotter middle diet, which was problem because she was a vegetarian. She would not eat red meat. I finally convinced her by asking her what she would do if it were a matter of life and death. She asked me if it was a matter of life and death. I said yes. She compromised. She would eat veal and eggs. Three days later, she called me back. I was a little nervous. I thought I might have given her the wrong diet, too hot as she was sixty years old, living in a very hot climate, etc. When I picked up the phone, she asked, "Is this the genius?" All her anxiety attacks had disappeared. She had been able to control them through diet and deep abdominal breathing. She also slept better and had great bowel movements

Atherosclerosis, arteriosclerosis

The arteries channel blood throughout the body. Blood (watery medium) carries nutrients, hormones, wastes, etc. to and from every cell, tissue. Protein and fat are thick, hard, sticky nutrients. **Too much**, especially animal, tends to thicken the blood (clots, high cholesterol) too much, which in turn thickens, pastes, clogs (plaque), narrows (atherosclerosis) and hardens the arteries (arteriosclerosis), stagnating and reducing overall blood, nutrient flow, especially to the extremities: head, arms and legs.

Long-term clogged arteries tend to cause headaches, insomnia, aneurisms, heart attacks and pain, inflammation, tension or numbness in the joints, bones, ligaments, muscles, etc. The colder middle diet is recommended, in addition to medical consultation.

Everything, including cholesterol and arterial plaque builds up and breaks down. Raw fruits and vegetables, bitter herbs naturally thin the blood, help dissolve and remove excess protein, fat, cholesterol, plaque, as does decreasing animal and fried foods. Many doctors recommend the vegetarian diet to their heart patients.

Arthritis

Arthritis is a generic term for inflammation (pain, swelling and redness) of the joint (where two or more bones join). Fluid sacs fill the joints spaces. Cartilage (gelatinous substance, shock absorber) caps, separates and cushions the ends of all movable bones. Ligaments hold the bones together. Tendons attach muscles to ligaments. Nerves, electrical impulses and blood (nutrients) stimulate, move, expand and contract, relax the muscles, tendons and ligaments, which move the bones according to their range of motion. Poor circulation via clogged arteries (hot), deficient blood (cold), injury, obesity (hot), etc. tends to cause arthritic pain.

There are three types of arthritis: (1) **rheumatoid** (autoimmune) (2) **gout** (excess uric acid) and (3) **osteo** (bone on bone). Chronic, long-term anemic, deficient blood, clogged arteries, obesity and or injury reduces blood, nutrient flow, especially to the extremities, arms and legs causing pain, dryness, swelling, inflammation, weakness, numbness, stiffness, Rheumatoid Arthritis, Peripheral Artery Disease, etc.

Protein and fat build thicken fuel and moisten. Long-term low protein, low fat and high carbohydrate diets tend to reduce, thin and weaken the blood. Thin, deficient, low protein, low fat blood, in the extreme, thins, dries, inflames, weakens and pains the muscles, tendons, nerves, etc. in the arms, legs, hands and feet. Too many cold, damp foods, drinks (ice cream, fruits, juices, cold drinks, sugar) dilute, weaken digestion, reduce nutrient absorption, and thin the blood.

Long-term high protein, high fat diets tend to thicken and the blood (clots, high cholesterol) and clog the arteries (plaque, atherosclerosis) stagnating and reducing circulation, especially to the extremities: head, arms and legs. Reduced circulation, blood, nutrients, dries, inflames, thins and pains the bones, ligaments, tendons, muscles, nerves causing arthritic symptoms (rheumatoid and psoriatic). Pain, numbness, while sitting or lying down with arms or legs crossed generally indicates clogged, narrow arteries.

High protein, high fat diets, in the extreme, also cause excessive **uric acid** (by-product of protein digestion) that can lodge in the joints (gout), in particular the big toe causing excruciating pain

Gout is more prevalent in western countries (high protein, high fat) and tends to attack men (high protein, fat diets) more than women (low protein, low fat).

Dietary cures for arthritis via blood deficiency and clogged arteries, depending on severity are relatively simple but time consuming, to rebuild and or cleanse the body. The hotter middle diet, more protein, fat, chicken, turkey, hard cheese, cooked foods, soups, vegetables, spices is recommended for "cold" arthritis.

The colder middle diet, meal plan is recommended for "hot" arthritis, thick blood, clogged arteries. Eat more cheese, nuts, seeds, vegetables (raw cabbage, celery) fruit (apples), spices (cumin, coriander, and fennel) and peppermint tea. Avoid alcohol and the nightshades (cooked tomatoes, potatoes, eggplant) which tend to worsen arthritic conditions.

Hot salves (contain hot herbs: camphor, capsicum/ cayenne pepper) used externally for reducing pain are also effective, especially when skin is wrapped, covered with plastic, which contains, drives heat down, into the skin, muscles, circulates blood. Glucosamine sulfate (1500 mg/ day) and bovine cartilage can help grow cartilage where there is cartilage. Check with your doctor first before using if you have an allergy to shellfish (source of GS).

Medication, blood thinners can also cause arthritic symptoms. Blood thinners thin the blood; remove excess protein, fat (cholesterol), which can thin the bones, muscles, skin, hair, nails, etc. Protein and fat builds, thickens all structure.

Diet and herbs cannot cure osteoarthritis (bone on bone). You cannot grow cartilage where there is none.

Case history: I used to suffer numbness and pain when I crossed my arms and legs, especially while sitting or lying down. I also suffered pain in my back and knees. I changed my diet, increased hard cheese, nuts, seeds fruits and vegetables (raw and cooked) while decreasing and or eliminating all animal food (except occasional turkey and chicken) and grain. My diet used to be one-third grain.

Within six months the pain, numbness, etc. in my arms and legs, disappeared, as long as I ate well. When I did not eat well, increased animal protein, fat and grain, the pain would return. Then, I would correct my diet and the pain would disappear, indicating that my circulation was getting better, despite the fact that I was getting older, nearing my sixtieth birthday. Everything (plaque, clots, etc.) builds up and breaks down.

Arthritis cold, deficient
Stage 1 Diet: long-term low protein, low fat, high carb
Stage 2 Digestion: abdominal bloating, gas
Stage 3 Elimination: loose stools, constipation
Stage 4 Blood deficiency: fatigue, pallor, coldness
Stage 5 Poor circulation: Rheumatoid Arthritis

Arthritis hot, overbuilt
Stage 1 Diet: long-term high protein, fat and starch
Stage 2 Digestion: abdominal bloating, gas
Stage 3 Elimination: constipation
Stage 4 Blood stagnation: clogged arteries, tension
Stage 5 Poor circulation: Rheumatoid Arthritis, gout
Stage 6 Psoriatic arthritis

Asthma

Asthma is a respiratory disorder caused by thick mucous in the lungs, bronchi and alveoli (where gas exchange occurs). Thick mucous tends to clog, obstruct the bronchi, alveoli, shortening the breath causing a wheezing cough (especially on the exhalation) and or expectoration of thick mucous. Extreme cold, damp diet or climate tends to cause thick mucous.

The lungs (includes throat, nose, sinuses and throat) are naturally moist.

Moisture, water facilitates the exchange of water-soluble gases (oxygen, carbon dioxide) between the lungs, blood (65% water) and environment. Too much or too little moisture tends to weaken the lungs, breath.

The body is naturally hot. Normal body temperature, heat (98.6°F) not only heats, protects but also regulates (thins) body fluids. Colder body temperatures thicken.

Long-term cold, damp diets, overexposure to cold, damp weather, A/C, living in a cold damp basement, etc. tend to lower body temperature, which cools, dampens the body in the same way the colder temperatures of nature harden water in the air into the morning dew, rain, snow or ice.

Colder body temperatures thicken fluids in the lungs, sinuses, throat, bronchi (passages), and alveoli into mucous and phlegm (thick mucous), that obstructs, shortens the breath: wheezing, sneezing, snoring, sinus infection and sleep apnea.

The digestive system, organs, 2- 3 meals per day, also heats, dries the body, especially the lungs. Digestive energy, heat naturally rises up into the lungs, throat and sinuses, drying, dissipating excess fluids. Protein and fat build fuel and heat. Long-term low protein, low fat diets weaken, cool the body (digestion, body temperature) as do too many cold damp foods (milk, ice cream, salads, tropical fruits, juices, cold drinks, etc.).

Excess cold, damp tends to attack women (cold, damp diets), children (undeveloped) and those living in cold, damp climates more than men (testosterone, high protein, fat diets). The hotter middle diet, spices, garlic (for cold, damp) is recommended.

Attention Deficit Disorder

Attention Deficit Disorder can have many causes: poor diet (low protein, low fat, high protein, high fat, sugar, etc.), overcrowded classrooms, lack of parental guidance, attention, etc. **Case History:** One of my customers came to see me about her eleven-year-old daughter (very thin) who had been diagnosed with ADD. Her school wanted to put her daughter on Ritalin in addition to the drugs that she was already taking: four months of Adderall and Dexedrine. She did not know what to do. I told her to bring her daughter in and let me question her. I had never counseled a child before but I did not think it would be any different from an adult, as the biology, choice of foods, etc. were the same. She brought her daughter in. I sat and questioned her. There was nothing wrong with her except for poor diet (too little protein) and lack of attention: home and school (overcrowded classrooms). I recommended more protein (red meat, eggs, chicken, turkey, etc.) especially for breakfast. She was already eating grains, cooked vegetables and fruits. I also advised fish liver oil in addition to greater personal attention.

Six months later, her mother wrote me a thank you letter, telling me how well her daughter was doing: recent report card, all A's and one B (math) without the use of Ritalin or any other drug.

Autoimmune Illnesses

The body is many structure functions that work together to produce greater structure and function. The immune system, digestion, circulation, respiration, etc. are not separate from blood, diet, environment, etc. Most autoimmune illnesses are cold, deficient, damp and tend to share similar symptoms, diets, gender, etc.

All disease progresses in **stages**, from one organ, symptom to another. Stage 1 is cause, which in general, is poor diet.

(1) **Long-term low protein, low fat** (milk, yogurt, cottage cheese, ice cream) and **high carbohydrate** (fruits, juices, cold drinks, sugar) diets weaken

(2) **Digestion**
- Abdominal bloating, pain, gas
- Nausea, vomiting, heartburn

(3) **Elimination**
- Loose stools, constipation

(4) **Blood**
- Anemia, fatigue, pallor, coldness

(5) **Circulation**
- Pain, inflammation, arthritis
- Mucous, phlegm, cysts
- Weak immunity

(6) **Organ**
- Leucorrhea, yeast infection, edema, cellulite
- Autoimmune disease

Weak, incomplete digestion increases abdominal bloating (small and large intestines) via an increase in waste product as all food, nutrients and non-nutrients not digested, absorbed become toxic waste that is moved down into the large intestine. Daily elimination is necessary; otherwise, re-absorption into the blood and lymph may occur; and in the extreme, cause autointoxication, weakening of the body's immune system increasing antibodies that attack healthy tissues and other body materials. The large intestine tends to be the breeding ground, not the cause of autoimmune illnesses.

Blood deficiency, reduced circulation tends to cause fatigue, pallor, pain, numbness, inflammation, rheumatoid arthritis, autoimmune illnesses, etc. Most autoimmune illnesses share similar symptoms.

Lupus: *abdominal pain*, weight loss, fatigue, skin rash, *nausea, vomiting, diarrhea* and *constipation*

Crohn's Disease: *pain* in abdomen, right lower quadrant, appendix, *diarrhea, nausea,* fever, *fatigue,* weight loss

Fibromyalgia: chronic, achy muscular *pain*, dizziness, *fatigue*, Irritable Bowel Syndrome (abdominal pain, bloating, gas, *diarrhea, constipation)* anorexia), CFS

Chronic Fatigue Syndrome (CFS): *extreme fatigue*, aching muscles, joints, headaches, low blood pressure, fever, loss of appetite, upper respiratory infections, nasal congestion, mucous, phlegm, Candidiasis, *loose stools, diarrhea, constipation,* depression, anxiety, etc.

Irritable Bowel Syndrome (IBS): *abdominal pain*, cramps, *loose stools, diarrhea, constipation*

Autoimmune illnesses in general tend to attack women (menstruation and tendency to eat low protein, low fat diets) more than men. This combination makes them more susceptible to weak digestion, elimination, blood deficiency, autoimmune illnesses, etc.

Autoimmune illnesses are chronic, long-lasting diseases taking time (months, years) to develop and cure. The hotter middle diet is recommended for cold, damp autoimmune diseases.

16

"B" Diseases

Blood (thick and thin)

Thick blood high protein, high fat
- Clots (thrombus), high cholesterol, uric acid
- Atherosclerosis, high blood pressure, chest pain
- Tumors, cancer, insomnia, dysmenorrhea
- Poor circulation, gout, arthritis
- Dry, scaly, oily skin, warts, psoriasis
- Dietary treatment: colder middle diet

Thin blood low protein, low fat
- Blood deficiency, fatigue, coldness, pallor
- Bruising, bleeding easily, poor circulation
- Arthritis (Rheumatoid), insomnia
- Infertility, miscarriage, impotence
- Osteoporosis, thin, cracked skin, eczema
- Dietary treatment: hotter middle diet

Blood type diet

There are four blood types: A, B, AB and O, each with a yin or yang nature. The blood type diet (eating for your blood type) is a constitutional medicine that lacks flexibility, may be opposite, contrary to one's condition. The vegetarian diet (low protein, low fat, cooling) is recommended for type A, which has a strong yang, pitta constitution and is great, beneficial for those suffering high protein, fat diseases or live in a hot climate but not appropriate for those suffering blood deficiency or living in a cold climate, which may require animal protein, flesh.

Blood Pressure

Blood pressure is the force of blood on the walls of the arteries produced by the contraction of the heart (left ventricle). Normal blood pressure is approximately **120/80**. Any reading sufficiently above or below indicates high (hypertension) or low (hypotension) blood pressure, and in the extreme, can damage the heart, brain, kidneys, etc. The force of blood is not only dependent on the heart and arteries, but also diet. Too much or too little protein, fat, in the extreme, thickens or thins the blood, arteries, too much, increasing or decreasing blood pressure.

High protein, high fat (red meat, chicken, fried foods, etc.) diets, in the extreme, thicken the blood (clots, high cholesterol) and arteries (plaque, atherosclerosis) increasing blood pressure.

Too much grain, especially processed (bread, crackers, cookies, chips) clogs and pastes the intestines, which adversely affect digestion, elimination, circulation, blood pressure as can tight belts, clothing, obesity and nervousness. Long-term high blood pressure eventually weakens the heart, causing low blood pressure.

The colder middle diet, less fat, less eating, more fruit, vegetables, bitter herbs (page 54) is recommended for all high protein, fat diseases (high cholesterol, high blood pressure, atherosclerosis, etc.) as is medical consultation.

Too little protein, fat, in the extreme, thins the blood, weakens the heart, circulation, decreasing blood pressure. It takes energy, fuel (protein, fat) to move the blood. The hotter middle diet is recommended, as is medical consultation.

Body Odor

The body is sweet and sour by nature. Blood, protein, fat and sugar are naturally sweet (taste, smell). Digestion (fermentation), sour foods (dairy) and grain tend to produce sour body odor. Animal, fried foods, overeating and disorderly eating, in the extreme, tend to produce **foul** body odor. Long-term cold, damp, low protein, low fat diets, weak digestion and obesity tend to produce sweet, sour and or **musty** body odor.

The stomach is the first digestive organ to receive and **process, mix food and fluids** with hydrochloric acid (**HCl**) and other enzymes, designed specifically to digest animal protein, fat. This mixture sits ferments (sours), breaks down before moving down into the small intestine, for further digestion, nutrient absorption. Digestion, fermentation is a souring process, which is why everyone tends to have a slightly sour smell. Food that spends too long of a time in the stomach tends to over ferment, spoil, creating an **excessive sour smell** that overflows, rises up and out the **throat, breath, armpits**, etc.

Long-term cold, damp diets, obesity, edema, cellulite, inactivity and or bulimia increase sweet, musty body odor. Too many fruits, juices, cold drinks dilute, weaken and slow elimination (loose stools, constipation). Excess waste, dampness and diabetes tend to produce **sweet, sour and or musty body odor**. The musty, sweet smell is a stale, moldy usually associated with long-term deficiency, dryness, stagnation, dampness and or deterioration.

Too many animal, fried foods, alcohol and ice cream increase hot, damp, greasy and smelly (offensively sweet odor) skin rashes (damp heat) in the armpits and groin.

The middle diet, meal plan adjusted accordingly is recommended. Cooked foods and spices increase digestion help drain dampness. *Bitter herbs* also drain dampness, but are very cooling: *contraindicated* for weak, cold digestion (source of dampness). Reduce dairy, grains, salads, cold drinks, alcohol, overeating, etc. It takes months and or years of good eating to eliminate and replace old, diseased tissues with new healthy smelling vibrant tissues.

Bones

Jing, protein, fat (especially animal) and minerals (calcium, phosphorus, etc.) build, thicken the bones. Long-term low protein, low fat (soft dairy) and high carbohydrate (salads, tropical fruits, juices, sugar, caffeine, cold drinks, etc.) diets, tend to thin the blood, which in turn, thins, weakens the bones. Americans, as a whole, consume more dairy products and calcium than any other country; yet have an extremely high osteoporosis rate, especially among women.

Chronic low protein, low fat blood, thins, dries and weakens the skin, hair, nails, bones (osteoporosis), immunity, reproduction (infertility, miscarriage), etc. Too many salads, fruits, juices, cold drinks, especially at the beginning of the meal weakens, decreases digestion, elimination and nutrient absorption, thins the blood, decreases protein, fat.

American women (low protein, low fat and high carbohydrate diets) tend to have a **high** osteoporosis rate despite consuming **high amounts** of dairy and calcium. The primary cause is not calcium and dairy deficiency but instead long-term blood, protein and fat (especially animal) deficiency. Menopause is also a cause.

Menopause represents a dual decline in estrogen and blood. The decline of estrogen and blood does weaken, gradually thin the bones, which is natural. However, it is the underlying blood deficiency, which is the real culprit.

Long-term blood, protein and fat deficiency **accelerates** premature aging, drying, thinning of bones, as does the lack of exercise. Exercise stimulates growth in the bones. Sedentary lifestyle dissolves. It is generally the chronically blood, protein and fat deficient, who tend to suffer severe osteoporosis, early menopause, hot flashes, etc.

The worst food for the bones is **caffeine** (coffee, black tea, colas, soft drinks, weight loss supplements, etc.). Caffeine in TCM is generally avoided as it over stimulates the adrenal glands and kidneys, production, burning of jing, hormones, youth, etc.

Jing (sexual essence) is the primary substance of the marrow, bones, brain, spine, nerves, etc. It is the fountain of youth (strong bones), when full and the specter of old age in decline. Excessive (daily) sex, coffee, caffeine and stimulants accelerate the decline of jing: thinning of the bones, skin, hair, nails, brain, sleep, memory, youth, etc.

The hotter middle diet for blood deficiency osteoporosis is recommended, in addition to calcium rich sources: seaweeds, sesame seeds (ground up), green vegetables (broccoli, cabbage, kale, and collards), horsetail and brewers yeast, which contain more calcium than dairy products. Fish oil supplements help strengthen the bones and nervous system. Reduce avoid coffee, caffeine and concentrated sweets. Both deplete minerals weaken the bones. Reduce or eliminate sex, masturbation.

Breast lumps, cancer

Most breast lumps are harmless **cysts** (abnormal fluid filled sacs, common in the breasts) that come and go, but can harden over time. Cysts are not cancerous, as they contain no protein or fat, unlike **tumors** (blood, protein, fat rich). Breast cancer is a firm, immovable cancerous lump, tumor. It attacks one in eight women, generally over the age of forty and is usually pain free. Normal fibrocystic changes during the menstrual cycle and or estrogen supplements promotes cellular growth in the breasts and reproductive organs may cause lumps that do not move.

Body temperature (98.6°F) heats, protects and dries (regulates, thins body fluids) the body. Digestion also heats and dries the body, especially the lungs, chest, (heat rises).

Cold condenses. Lower body temperatures via long-term blood deficiency and weak digestion cool and harden water in the lungs, sinuses, breasts, etc. into mucous, phlegm, cysts, lumps, in the same way colder temperatures cool, harden water in the air, on the ground into rain, snow and ice. Long-term cold, damp low protein, fat diets weaken and cool the body.

Most lumps although harmless and normal should be checked, monitored regularly via physical examination. Know all your options, and do not hesitate to self examine and or question your daily diet.

The hotter middle diet, meal plan, more beans, cooked foods, spices, etc. for breast lumps, cysts is recommended. Cooked foods, soups, spices and bitter herbs (dandelion) help eliminate excess moisture.

Breast cancer, like most cancers, comes in the form of a tumor. All tumors are blood, protein and fat rich. Protein and fat build, fuel all structure, function, including tumors and cancer. No one has ever developed cancer from eating too many fruits and vegetables. Incidences of cancer (breast, colon and prostate) are highest in America, Argentina and other countries with high animal protein, fat diets.

Cancer is a disorder of unrestrained cellular growth. **Estrogen** supplements, animal protein, fat, processed foods, smoking and stimulant drugs feed and accelerate the growth of cancer. Early menstruation prior to age ten or menopause after age fifty-five can also be a cause. Avoid caffeine, as it is a known breast irritant. The colder middle diet (and medical consultation) is recommended.

While there is "no cure for cancer", some people have cured. Everything builds up and breaks down. Cancer in tumor form can be starved, broken down via low protein, low fat (vegetarian), raw vegetables, spices, fruit and herbs (Essiac tea). Cancer is a deadly disease that requires medical consultation, and or treatment, as radiation and or removal may be the best option. A yellow, bloody or clear discharge from the nipple generally indicates cancer of the breast.

Bronchitis

Bronchitis is inflammation or obstruction in the bronchial tubes (connects throat, trachea, windpipe to the lungs, alveoli). The lungs, bronchi, alveoli (small air sacs where gas exchange occurs) are naturally moist (water, mucous, blood) which facilitates the exchange of water-soluble gases (oxygen and carbon dioxide).

Too much moisture (mucous, phlegm) and or contaminants (smoke, pollution, etc.) tend to obstruct and inflame the bronchi, shortening the breath while also providing the **breeding ground for bacterial and viral infections**.

Excess water, mucous, phlegm tends to clog the bronchi, alveoli reducing oxygen exchange, obstructing and shortening the breath

- Coughing, panting (to take in more oxygen)
- Sore throat, fever, fatigue
- Pain in the chest
- Sudden chills, shaking
- Inflammation of the bronchi, bronchospasm

Lower body temperatures via long-term blood deficiency cool harden water in the lungs, sinuses, breasts, etc. into mucous, phlegm, cysts, etc. Long-term cold, damp diets (soft dairy, juices, cold drinks, etc.) cool, dampen the body.

The hotter middle diet, meal plan, **less** animal, fish, egg, dairy, nuts, seeds, raw fruits, juices and grains (wheat, rice) and **more** beans, cooked vegetables (lightly boiled, steamed), mushrooms, and hot spices for cold, damp bronchitis is recommended. Cooked foods, soups, spices, mushrooms, etc. increase digestion and dry dampness: mucous, phlegm, cysts, loose stools, etc. in conjunction with a decrease in cold drinks, ice cream, fruit juices, soda, sugar, etc. Antibiotics and bitter herbs (laxatives) are cold in nature. Check with your doctor.

17

"C" Diseases

Cancer

Cancer is abnormal malignant growth of cells that invade and spread (metastasize) to other tissues. It generally occurs, starts in the form of a tumor (stagnant blood) then deteriorates, turns malignant. All tumors are blood, protein and fat rich. Long-term high animal protein, fat, diets, smoking and other carcinogens tend to cause cancer. The U.S. and Argentina the two largest consumers of animal flesh have the highest cancer rates (prostate, colon, etc.).

The colder middle diet (**raw beets**) is recommended, as is medical consultation. Chemotherapy is a common treatment for cancer. The chemical drugs used to kill cancer also poison, kill healthy tissues, which is why they must quickly be eliminated, cleansed from the body, once treatment ends. Vegetable soups with spices and seaweeds, and baths (with salt or seaweed) help cleanse, eliminate toxic chemicals from the body.

Candidiasis

Candidiasis is a yeast-like infection caused by the proliferation of normally occurring yeast-like fungus that tends to attack women (key symptom). It tends to be a cold, damp pathology caused by long-term low protein, low fat, cold, damp diet, antibiotics, infection and or chronic illness. Many women tend to eat cold, damp diets.

Primary symptoms: Thrush, white spots on tongue or inside the mouth, cheeks; skin rash, fungal infections and itching, toenail and fingernail fungus, and vaginitis, yeast infections, discharges, etc.

Secondary symptoms: Abdominal pain, heartburn, bad breath, loose stools, diarrhea, constipation, colitis, rectal itching, headaches, PMS, cough, sore throat, clogged nose and sinuses, extreme fatigue, muscle and joint pain, numbness, tingling in the extremities, arthritis, memory loss, mood swings, kidney and bladder infections and or prostatitis.

All disease progresses in stages. (1) Poor diet tends to weaken and slow (2) digestion and (3) elimination providing the damp, moist breeding ground for cold, damp (watery, gooey) diseases: bacterial infection, fungi, thrush, diaper, groin rash, fungus, yeast infections, Candidiasis, etc. The "secondary" symptoms predate the primary symptoms of Candidiasis.

Long-term **cold, damp, diets** (cottage cheese, milk, ice cream, salads, juices, sodas, cold drinks, sugar) cool, weaken, moisten and slow **digestion and elimination**

- Abdominal pain, heartburn, bad breath
- Loose stools, diarrhea, constipation
- Colitis, rectal itching

They also thin weaken the **blood**, body, causing

- Muscle and joint pain, extreme fatigue, numbness
- Tingling in the extremities, headaches and coldness

Body temperature (98.6°F), digestion and sunshine heats, dries, regulates, thins body fluids, especially in the lungs, chest, throat, sinuses, vagina and uterus.

Long-term blood, protein and fat deficiency, chronic illness and or overexposure to **cold, damp** weather lowers body temperature, which cools and hardens bodily fluids in the same way the cold temperatures of nature cool harden water in the air, into rain, snow and ice. **Colder body temperatures** increase, thicken fluids:

Lungs, sinuses and throat
- Mucous, phlegm, sore throat
- Shortness of breath, sinusitis, sleep apnea

Mouth
- Thrush, white spots on tongue

Cheeks
- Rashes, itching

Large intestine
- Candidiasis

Uterus, vagina
- White vaginal discharges, vaginitis, yeast infection

Toes, fingernails
- Fungus

In Ayurveda, there are three types of Candida Albicans: vata, pitta and kapha.

- **Kapha** symptoms include mucous, phlegm, edema, swollen glands, frequent colds and flu, heaviness, etc. Long-term cold, damp diets tend to produce kapha.

- **Vata** symptoms also include insomnia, restlessness, nervousness, lower back pain and dry skin, fatigue, shaking and ringing in the ears. Long-term low protein, fat diets produce vata.

- **Pitta** symptoms include heartburn, hyperacidity, burning sensation, fever and thirst. Long-term high protein, fat diets produce pitta.

Candida Albicans is generally a cold damp disease. For more information please read **Ayurvedic Healing** by Dr. David Frawley, O.M.D.

The **hotter middle diet** is recommended in general for vata kapha conditions. **The colder middle diet** is recommended for pitta kapha conditions.

- **Spices and bitter herbs** (golden seal, barberry root) drain dampness (fluids, yeast) and are antibacterial, antifungal, etc. Bitter herbs are cold in nature and used sparingly if digestion is weak
- **Black and white fungus** dry, drain excess dampness in the lungs, vagina and intestines, help constipation and hypertension. Many Asian women eat fungi (includes mushrooms) regularly and do not develop yeast infections, unlike their American counterparts who eat little or no fungi.
- **Pau d'arco tea** also dries damp.
- Avoid sugar and dairy (cold, damp).
- Check with your doctor first before using.

Candidiasis
- Stage 1: Poor diet (cold, damp, deficient)
- Stage 2: Indigestion (abdominal bloating, gas)
- Stage 3: Poor elimination (diarrhea, constipation)
- Stage 4: Blood deficiency (fatigue, pain, pallor)
- Stage 5: Poor circulation (coldness, mucous)
- Stage 6: Candidiasis, yeast infections, vaginitis

Cellulite

Cellulite is excess water and fat that accumulates in pockets around the abdomen and thighs, more so in women than men. Many women tend to eat cold, damp diets (milk, yogurt, cottage cheese, ice cream, salads, tropical fruits, juices, cold drinks, ice water, etc.).

Cold, damp, anemic (low protein, low fat) diets, overeating and late meals, snacks tend to cool, moisten and weaken digestion and elimination causing abdominal bloating, loose stools; and in the extreme, edema, cellulite, anemia, etc.

Strong digestion is the ultimate fat and water burner as it breaks down, burns excess protein, fat, water, etc.

- **Protein and fat** build fuel digestion. Low protein, low fat diets, in the extreme, weaken digestion.

- **Water, minerals, sugar** reduce, cleanse, cool and moisten. Too many salads, vegetables, fruits (citrus, tropical), juices, cold drinks and refined sugars tend to weaken and or dilute digestion, acid, enzymes.

Weak digestion burns less fat and water, storing more (mucous, phlegm, cysts, edema and cellulite) in the chest, lungs, arms, hips, and or thighs.

Cellulite is generally a cold, damp condition, caused by long-term cold, damp, low protein, low fat (milk, yogurt, cottage cheese, ice cream, etc.) diet. The **hotter** middle diet (lesser animal, nuts and oil) is recommended. Beans, cooked foods, soups, spices (cumin, fennel, ginger, cayenne, turmeric, etc.) increase digestion, burning of excess fluids, fat. Reduce cold, damp foods: milk, ice cream, grains, salads, tropical fruits, juices, cold drinks, sugar. Avoid big dinners and late night eating, snacks.

Bitter herbs (golden seal, gentian, aloe vera, barberry, Swedish Bitters, etc.) also drain excess fat, water, cellulite, but are contraindicated when digestion and elimination (loose stools) are cold, damp. The bitter taste is cold, drying.

Exercise increases metabolism. You do not need to join a gym, club to walk. Cellulite takes months, years to develop and consequently months plus to cure.

Cholesterol

Saturated fat, commonly found in animal foods, is high in cholesterol. Cholesterol (fatty substance) is an essential part of every cell, tissue, including the brain and nervous system. Too much or too little, in the extreme tends to cause disease.

Saturated fat, in the extreme, increases
- Blood cholesterol
- Low-density lipoproteins (LDL)
- Very low-density lipoproteins (VLDL)

LDL and VLDL carry and harden cholesterol into plaque that binds to the interior walls of the arteries, decreasing size, diameter. Excess protein thickens the blood into clots (thrombus).

Plaque and clots obstruct and reduce the flow of blood, within the arteries. Clogged and narrow arteries stagnate and reduce circulation, blood, especially to the extremities: head, arms and legs: insomnia, dizziness, pain, inflammation, weakness, numbness, etc.

Unsaturated fatty acids (beans, nuts and seeds), increase the number of high-density lipoproteins (HDL) which remove and transport cholesterol back to the liver, where it is transformed into bile salts, and passed into the bowels. Too many unsaturated fatty acids lessen HDL.

All blood passes though the liver. The liver stores, cleanses (removes excess protein, fat, cholesterol, uric acid) and releases the blood.

Too much animal protein, fat, in the extreme, clogs and weakens the liver. Less protein, fat, cholesterol are cleansed, removed, more stays in the blood (clots, high cholesterol), arteries, skin (acne, psoriasis).

Weak digestion via overeating, blood deficiency, caffeine, alcohol, sugar and stress also increases cholesterol. High cholesterol is only a problem when it starts to collect. Once it has collected, it is difficult, but not impossible to remove.

The **colder middle diet**, meal plan (page 54- 55) vegetables raw and cooked, bitter herbs and mild spices, garlic, beans, nuts (walnuts), seeds and grains for high cholesterol are recommended. Reduce or eliminate animal food. The less animal fat you eat, the less cholesterol, VLDL and LDL produced and the more cleansed, removed from the arteries, thighs, hips, brain, etc. Snack on fruits especially during the night. Avoid alcohol, overeating and late night eating. The body will clean itself of excess, when given the chance.

Spices increase digestion, burning of excess fat, water, etc. Bitter herbs (golden seal, gentian, aloe vera, green tea and chrysanthemum tea) help digest, eliminate excess cholesterol, fat. Bitter herbs are contraindicated for cold, damp digestion. Too many dries the blood.

Blood pressure lowering medications and or thinning agents may lower pressure, prevent new build up, but not necessarily eliminate old build up. It is the old build up you have to eliminate to cure clogged arteries.

Long-term low protein, low fat diets tend to cause low cholesterol, thin blood weakening the heart, brain, nervous system, bones, muscles, etc.

Pain in the arms and legs when resting is a general symptom of poor circulation via clogged arteries or blood deficiency (thin blood).

Chronic Fatigue Syndrome (CFS)

The following are symptoms of CFS:

- Extreme fatigue, aching muscles and joints
- Headaches, low blood pressure
- Fever, loss of appetite, constipation, diarrhea
- Mucous, phlegm, nasal congestion
- Upper respiratory infections
- Candidiasis, depression
- Tends to attack women more than men

All of the symptoms, including the name, indicate extreme deficiency and coldness. (1) Long-term cold, damp, low protein, low fat and high carbohydrate diets tend to weaken (2) digestion, (3) elimination, (4) blood, (5) circulation, body temperature, immunity and (6), autoimmune illnesses, CFS.

Lower body temperatures via long-term blood deficiency or chronic illness cools and hardens fluids in the lungs, throat, sinuses and nose into mucous, phlegm: coughing, shortness of breath, inflammation, bacterial infections, etc., in the same way colder temperatures cool, harden moisture in the air, into the morning dew, rain, snow, etc

Many women tend to eat cold, damp, low protein, low fat (soft dairy) and high carbohydrate (bread, salads, tropical fruits, juices, smoothies, shakes, cold drinks, ice water, sugar) diets. The hotter middle diet for cold, damp is recommended. More info: autoimmune illnesses (172)

Circulation

The heart commands, controls circulation of blood via its system of vessels: arteries, veins and capillaries. Blood carries nutrients and wastes to and from every cell. **Protein and fat** build, fuel. (1) Too much (especially animal) or (2) too little reduces circulation, blood flow, especially to the extremities: arms and legs producing arthritic symptoms (pain, weakness, dryness, inflammation, numbness, etc.). (3) Too much grain, especially processed also decreases circulation.

The liver stores, cleanses (removes excess protein, fat, cholesterol) and releases the blood. **Too much** animal protein, fat tends to clog, weaken the liver. Less protein, fat is removed; more stays, collects and

- Thickens the blood (clots, high cholesterol)

- Thick blood in the extreme tends to clog and narrow the arteries (plaque, atherosclerosis). Clogged arteries reduce blood flow, especially to the extremities, head, arms and legs:

- Poor memory, dizziness, insomnia, seizure, stroke, pain, arthritis, Restless Leg Syndrome (RLS), metacarpal syndrome, etc

Too little protein and fat, in the extreme, thins and weakens the blood, circulation, heart, etc.

- Chronically thin (deficient) blood tends to cause

- Pain, inflammation, numbness, etc., in arms and legs (especially when lying down)

- Pale complexion (pallor), pale, dry tongue.

Too much grain, especially processed (bread, noodles, cookies, pretzels, chips, etc.) tends to clog the small and large intestines, which also reduces circulation.

The middle diet adjusted accordingly is recommended. Reduce processed grains. Bitter herbs (contraindicated for cold, damp, weak conditions) and spices (cinnamon) help eliminate excess protein, fat, cholesterol, increase circulation.

Poor circulation cold, deficient
Stage 1 Diet: long-term low protein, low fat, high carb
Stage 2 Digestion: abdominal bloating, gas
Stage 3 Elimination: loose stools
Stage 4 Blood deficiency: pain, inflammation
Stage 5 Poor circulation: Rheumatoid Arthritis, RLS

Poor circulation hot, overbuilt
Stage 1 Diet: long-term high protein, fat, starch
Stage 2 Digestion: abdominal bloating, gas
Stage 3 Elimination: constipation,
Stage 4 Blood stagnation: tension, pain, inflammation
Stage 5 Poor circulation: arthritis, gout, RLS

Cirrhosis

Cirrhosis is a chronic (long-term) condition of the liver in which fibrous tissue and nodules replace healthy tissue disrupting blood flow and function. Cirrhosis is common among alcoholics. Alcohol is very drying as well as damaging to the brain (kills brain cells).

- Nausea, severe abdominal bloating
- Light colored stools, short temper
- Tight gripping in the right side below and behind right rib cage

It is important to drink a lot of water when consuming alcohol. The colder middle diet, elimination of alcohol in addition to medical consultation is recommended.

Cold hands and feet

The heart pumps the blood via the arteries, veins and capillaries to all structure function. The entire body is warmed, nourished by blood. Blood carries nutrients, especially protein and fat, which build, thicken, fuel and heat. Chronic blood deficiency via long-term low protein, low fat and high carbohydrate diets and or excessive sex tends to cause cold hands, cold feet.

Blood, protein and fat deficiency reduces, thins all structure, function producing: coldness, pain, inflammation, weakness, numbness, shaking, dizziness, etc. It takes a certain amount of fuel, energy, protein and fat to heat the whole body, depending on climate. Chicken, turkey, eggs, hard cheese contain more protein, fat, than soft dairy (milk, yogurt and soft cheese), beans, nuts, etc. Too many fruits, juices, cold drinks weaken the body.

Occasional coldness in the hands and feet is normal, especially during the winter as blood naturally rushes back to the chest and abdomen to protect and nourish the vital organs, which leaves the extremities, hands, feet and head with less blood, nutrients, warmth, etc. causing them to become cold, weak, shaky, numb, inflamed, etc.

The hotter middle diet is recommended, as is exercise, walking, 20+ minutes 1-2 times per day (increases circulation, warmth). Lose weight as obesity reduces circulation. Lasting, persistent coldness is abnormal, chronic requiring medical consultation +/- treatment.

Common Cold and Flu

The common cold and flu are respiratory diseases caused by viruses. Both are acute in nature.

The common cold primarily affects the nose, throat and sinuses producing

- Runny nose, watery eyes and sore throat

The flu is a deeper cold, viral infection in the respiratory tract producing

- Fever, sore throat, cough, headache, muscle aches, fatigue

Most people catch cold because they are **cold, weak**. The body is naturally warm; hot (98.6°F), which protects the body against colds, flu. Lower body temperatures via anemic diet, cold climate, chronic illness, etc, predispose, invites one to catch, develop the common cold, flu.

Body temperature (98.6°F), digestion, protein, fat, spices and sunshine heats (kills bacteria, viruses), protects, and dries the body. Too little protein and fat thins the blood, cools the body. Too many cold, damp, foods, drinks: milk, yogurt, soft cheese, ice cream, tropical fruits, juices, smoothies, cold drinks and sugar decreases digestion, blood and body temperature.

Colder body temperatures tend to cool, slow and dampen the body, lungs, throat, ears, sinuses and nose with excess fluids (mucous, phlegm), in the same way, colder temperatures cool, slow and harden water in the air, into rain, snow and ice.

Excess fluids, mucous, phlegm obstructs the nasal passages

- Coughing, sneezing, snoring, hacking
- Runny nose, sore throat
- Provide breeding ground for bacteria, viruses

Colder temperatures also drain blood from the extremities, head, arms and legs: cold, weak, numb, and shaky, trembling.

Digestive symptoms (abdominal bloating, gas) are the key factor in determining whether the cause is internal, dietary or external (winter, A/C, etc.). An external, environmental attack initially does not produce any digestive disturbances, symptoms.

Long-term low protein fat diets also weaken the lungs, respiration and the skin, opening and closing of the pores, which controls external immunity (Wei chi). Closed pores retain energy, heat while preventing external invasion of environmental cold, heat, dampness, etc. Open pores dissipate excess internal energy, heat (cool the body), but can also allow entry of external pathogens

The body generally produces a fever, whenever it catches, becomes cold. Fever, higher body temperatures heat and dry excessive cold, damp in addition to killing certain bacteria and viruses.

All flu's (acute, contagious) are viral in nature and vary in strength, as does the individual. Not everyone gets sick when "attacked" by a pathogenic virus, as some have better immune systems. The healthier, warmer you become, the less chance that you will catch, develop the common cold, flu. Athletes and the active in general, due to increased physical activity, catch fewer colds.

The hotter middle diet, animal protein, fat, cooked foods, spices (page 56), exercise and sexual moderation strengthen the immune system, digestion, etc. Spices heat the body, perspiration, increase and dry dampness.

The common cold, if treated day one or two, is easy to cure. Increase hot soups, spices, protein, fat, extra clothing, hot baths, sweating, etc. while reducing all cold, damp foods, drinks. Peppermint tea helps moisten dry, sore throats, counter coughing. Vitamin C, golden seal and echinacea combination are also effective in curing the common cold, when taken at the onset. Flu's are more difficult to cure, requiring medical attention.

Constipation

Constipation is infrequent and or dry stools that are difficult to pass. It can have hot (too much protein, fat, hot spices) and cold (low protein, fat, bitter herbs, processed grains, sedentary lifestyle) causes.

The stools are made from food (nutrients, non-nutrients, fiber) and bacteria. Protein and fat build thicken and dry. Water, minerals, fruits, vegetables, moisten and loosen. Too much protein, fat, grain, hot spices, smoking, coffee and alcohol or too little fruit, vegetables tend to dry, harden and slow the stools, create diverticulitis (pockets), polyps, tumors, etc. which also slow the stools.

Too little protein, fat and or too many fruits, juices, sodas, cold drinks weaken peristalsis, wave-like contractions of muscles within the small intestine, which help push food down into the large intestine, slowing and or stagnating the stools. Too little exercise, sedentary lifestyle, sitting or lying down after eating also weakens elimination, causes constipation.

Exercise and deep abdominal breathing increases peristalsis via movement of the diaphragm (muscular partition divides the chest from the abdomen). The diaphragm moves up and down as the lungs expand and contract, which massages the intestines, increasing peristalsis, downward movement.

The middle diet, meal plan, adjusted accordingly is recommended. Eat a light, early dinner, as late night meals, increases constipation.

Deficiency constipation
- Flax seeds benefit deficiency conditions, but worsen aggravate pitta, high protein, high fat.

Dry constipation
- 1 TB of olive or sesame oil in cooking

- Black or white fungus or mushrooms (moistening, mucilaginous, slide easily through the intestines). Check with your doctor, as some people have allergies to fungus and certain herbs.

- Psyllium seeds, husks (bulk, lubricating laxative) 2TB in two 16 oz. glasses of water, two times per day

- Bran (too much leaches calcium) and or rhubarb

Crohn's Disease

Crohn's Disease (stage 6) is a chronic inflammatory condition of the large (cecum to rectum) or small intestine (end part) producing abdominal pain, nausea, diarrhea, weakness, fever and or weight loss. It tends to attack children (underdeveloped) more than adults.

Poor diet (overeating, too much protein, fat, oil, bread, noodles, cookies, pastries, desserts, sugar, cold drinks, sodas, etc.) in the extreme tends to cause autoimmune illnesses (page 172- 4) especially in children, young adults and women (weak digestion and or tendency to eat cold, damp diets).

Poor diet tends to weaken, slow

- Digestion (abdominal bloating, gas)
- Elimination (loose stools, diarrhea)
- Nutrient absorption, blood
- Circulation

Producing:

- Weakness, fever, weight loss
- Inflammation, ulcers in the colon (ulcerative colitis)
- Autoimmune illnesses, Crohn's Disease

Proper diet can cure, depending on severity, discipline, etc. The middle diet, meal plan adjusted accordingly is recommended. Reduce avoid red meat, soft dairy, grains, nuts, oil, raw foods and sugar. Cooked foods are easy to digest.

18

"D" Diseases

Depression

Depression is a dejected, negative state, choice of mind that tends to affect women twice as much as men. There are two kinds of depression: unipolar and bipolar.

- **Unipolar**: depressive episodes occur several times throughout a person's life.
- **Bipolar**, also known as manic-depressive, starts out as depression but progresses into alternate periods of depression and mania.

The following are general symptoms of depression:

- Tendency to withdraw, hide from society
- Declining interest in pleasure and hobbies
- Feelings of worthlessness
- Chronically sad depressed, angry, irritable
- Thoughts of death or no emotion at all

Depression can have physical and mental causes. Some people become mentally depressed when their physical energy, blood, stools, weight, etc stagnates becomes stuck (obesity, constipation, injury, etc.). Negative thoughts, fixation on bad, painful events, relationships, etc. can also stagnate and depress the mind. Relief occurs once the blockage is removed. Proper diet, exercise, sunshine, etc. help move stagnant energy, relieve depression, but ultimately it is attitude, choice that determines happiness, sadness, depression, anger, etc.

Long-term cold, damp, low protein, low fat diets, overeating, and or excessive sex decreases energy, weakens and stagnates the body. Protein and fat build, fuel, heat. It takes energy, heat, stimulation (fueled by protein, fat, exercise, etc.) to move stagnant energy. Cooked foods and spices heat stimulate, move energy. Raw foods and soft dairy cool, dampen, but may also cleanse, remove blockages (constipation, tumors, etc.).

Low protein, low fat (especially soft dairy) and high carbohydrate (especially salads, fruits, juices, sugar and cold drinks) diets, weaken digestion. Digestion **transforms** food into blood. Chronically weak digestion reduces not only blood (energy) but also the ability to change, transform and move on.

Many women tend to cold, damp, low protein, low fat and high carbohydrate diets. They also menstruate. Menstruation drains blood, energy. It is hard to be happy, confident, male or female when losing blood, hemorrhaging 5- 7 days every month for thirty years. The combination of menstruation and cold, damp, low protein, low fat diets predispose women towards depression.

The seasons adjust are also a factor, as climate (sunny, cloudy, hot, cold, dry, wet, etc.) adjusts (speeds up, slows down, raises, sinks, increases, decreases, etc.) the flow of energy within the body

Depression is more prevalent during the fall, winter, cloudy, rainy days: when there is lesser light, energy and greater cold, dampness. **Happiness** is more prevalent during the day, spring and summer when there is more sun, light, energy, heat, stimulation. People, in general, are more depressed in Seattle, WA (damp, cloudy) than in Phoenix, AZ (hot, dry, and sunny).

Depression is also a function of **three neurotransmitters** (dopamine, serotonin and nor-epinephrine), that chemically affect the mind, mood.

- Serotonin (produced by the amino acid, tryptophan) eases tension, relaxes and calms the mind. Low levels of serotonin may lead to depression, anxiety and sleep disorder. Complex carbohydrates and turkey are high in tryptophan.
- Dopamine and norephidrine stimulate. Animal foods increase dopamine and nor-epinephrine.

The mind ultimately decides how one reacts to life's challenges, highs and lows by attaching positive or negative emotions, feelings, happiness, sadness, depression, anger, etc. to each individual event, person, job, relationships, etc. Negative emotions, reactions rarely accomplish anything. Most often they worsen, hurt, although sometimes provides the necessary spark, stimulus to change for the better.

Everyone has the same choice to act positively, turn the other cheek or react poorly, battle hate with hate, instead of love. True bliss, happiness, end of depression happens when you take a positive attitude that everything always works out for the best. Every thought, action is battle between being good (intelligence) and bad (ignorance). Reading uplifting spiritual books, doing good deeds is the best medicine. A healthy lifestyle (diet, exercise, meditation, etc.) also helps.

Modern medicine tends to treat depression chemically with stimulants, amphetamines. Ritalin (amphetamine) is commonly prescribed for children suffering A.D.D. Stimulants drugs heat, energize, stimulate, move as do cooked foods, exercise, sunshine, spices bright colors (red, orange, yellow) and inspiration.

Detoxification

The food we eat, the air we breathe and water we drink are generally tainted, poisoned with chemical preservatives, dyes, pollutants, etc., which poisons the body (organs, blood, etc.), as does weak digestion. Weak digestion (caused by poor diet, overeating, drugs, etc.) increases waste product as whatever food, nutrients, and non-nutrients, not digested, absorbed becomes waste. All waste, especially animal protein and fat is poisonous, which is why daily elimination is necessary, otherwise poisons can leach back into the bloodstream, organs, etc. Detoxification via dietary changes, herbs, exercise, sweating, etc. helps cleanse, eliminate toxins.

There are three ways to detox.

- **Stop** eating toxins and let the body clean itself.

- **Use cold,** cleansing, bitter herbs, minerals, etc. to detox, cleanse hot, overbuilt conditions (high cholesterol, high blood pressure, atherosclerosis, tumors, cancer, psoriasis, gout, etc.)

- **Use excess heat** (sweating, spices) to detox, cleanse drugs from the body.

Cold detoxification programs, formulas use bitter herbs (golden seal, gentian root and aloe vera), bulking, cleansing agents (psyllium), minerals (clay), acidophilus, digestive enzymes, spices, etc. Bitter herbs are cold, dry. They contract and move blood through the heart, arteries, liver, etc., help reduce cholesterol and fatty deposits, drain excess moisture, dampness (water, mucous, phlegm, cellulite, etc.) but are contraindicated for cold, deficient conditions: weak digestion and elimination, anemia, emaciation, etc.

Psyllium husks and clay (minerals) are cooling, moistening and cleansing. They **absorb and remove** water, impurities (toxins, chemicals, etc.), excess protein, fat, oil, flour, paste in the small and large intestines, and **contraindicated** for **cold, damp** and or **dry** conditions:

- Loose stools, mucous, phlegm, cysts
- Edema, cellulite
- Yeast infections, Candidiasis
- Thin, dry skin, hair and nails

Raw and cooked vegetables, seaweeds (salty, cold), black fungus (cold), etc. also clean the intestines, remove excess debris, paste.

Too many bitters, laxatives, psyllium and clay in combination with milk, yogurt, ice cream, tropical fruits, salads, and cold drinks cool, dampen and weaken digestion, which in turn, increases waste product as whatever food, fluids, nutrients and non-nutrients, not digested, absorbed, becomes waste. All waste especially protein and fat is toxic.

Detoxification always starts with the diet. Reduce eliminate the source of toxins.

- Impure, highly processed foods are highly toxic.

- Too much protein, fat tends to poison and clog the blood, liver, heart, arteries, intestines, etc.

- Too much flour pastes the intestines.

- Too many fruits weaken digestion and elimination.

- Overeating weakens digestion, increases toxins in the blood, organs, etc.

Digestive enzymes (hot) and **spices** (hot, drying) not only increase digestion and nutrient absorption but also counter the cold, damp nature of bitter herbs, psyllium and minerals.

Detoxification in general benefits the strong, overbuilt, not the weak, cold, which need to build, supplement. Spring and summer (excess energy, heat) are the best times to detox, and fall, winter, the worst as you may catch a cold if you detox (cool, cleanse) in the winter.

Cure disease with health. Building health prevents and cures disease. Disease cannot live, prosper unless you feed it. Like health, it has a specific but flexible diet. The body will heal itself when given the chance via correct diet, exercise, etc. It will also get sick when given the chance, wrong diet. Feed health, not disease. The middle diet, adjusted accordingly is recommended.

Diabetes

There are two kinds of diabetes: diabetes insipidus and diabetes mellitus. Diabetes mellitus (more common) is a chronic, complex metabolic disorder due to partial or total lack of insulin or the inability of insulin to function normally causing excessive urination, thirst, weight loss and excessive sugar in the blood or urine. Adult diabetes and blood sugar problems, in general are a function of diet. Type 1 (juvenile diabetes) is genetically predisposed. The first step to preventing and or curing diabetes (depending on severity) is changing diet.

The pancreas (Islets of Langerhans) secretes insulin and glucagon. **Insulin** lowers blood sugar (glucose) when it is too high, by converting it into **glycogen** (stored in the liver and muscles).

Glucagon converts glycogen in the liver back into glucose and released back into the bloodstream, which raises blood sugar. **Insulin lowers, glucagon raises**.

The level of blood sugar is a function of diet. **Simple sugars** (white, brown, natural, fruit, etc.) absorb directly into the bloodstream instantly raising blood sugar levels, while **grains** (complex sugars, polysaccharides) gradually increase. Increased blood sugar levels cause the pancreas to secrete insulin. Low blood sugar levels cause it top secrete glucagon.

Too many sweets: sugar, ice cream, cookies, alcohol, sodas, etc. excessively stimulate, overwork, weaken the pancreas, Islets of Langerhans, eventually decreasing insulin and glucagon production causing hypoglycemia, hyperglycemia and or diabetes (produces sweet body odor).

The pancreas (gland) is also a digestive organ (secretes digestive enzymes). Too much protein, fat and overeating, in the extreme, overworks, weakens the pancreas not only decreasing digestive enzymes but also insulin and glucagon, in addition to forming tumors, cancer in the pancreas, liver, etc. Too little protein, fat in the extreme, also weakens the pancreas, digestion.

Low protein, low fat diets tend to weaken the body, thereby increasing sugar cravings and overeating for al quick energy boost, while well-balanced diets leave one satisfied, with little or no cravings. Vegetables and fruits are not only high in vitamins, fiber, but also sugar, which helps satisfy the sweet taste. Too little, fruit, vegetables in the diet tends to cause sugar cravings, overeating. Bitter herbs (golden seal, turmeric, aloe vera, barberry, etc.) help regulate sugar and fat metabolism.

The hotter middle diet is recommended for diabetes caused by deficiency, emaciation via low protein, low fat and high sugar diet. The colder middle diet, bitter herbs is recommended for diabetes caused by excess, obesity via high protein, fat, starch and sugar. Sweet vegetables (carrots, parsnips, hard squash, etc.) stimulate, nourish the spleen, pancreas in addition to Siberian Ginseng. Many people have cured diabetes, gotten off insulin.

Diarrhea

Diarrhea (frequent or loose stools) has many causes: poor diet, indigestion, contaminated water, bacterial infection, drugs, spoiled foods, caffeine, magnesium supplements, laxatives, antibiotics, excessive alcohol, inflammatory bowel disease, ulcerative colitis, IBS, Crohn's Disease, etc. It is generally treated with diet, herbs and or drugs.

The body digests, transforms food, nutrients into blood. Whatever food, nutrients, not digested, absorbed becomes waste, sent moved down into the large intestine, for eventual elimination. Building nutrients and grains thicken; paste the stools Cleansing foods moisten, thin.

Normal, healthy stools are banana shaped, firm and relatively odorless. Unhealthy stools are loose, dry, frequent, infrequent, constipated and stinky.

Water, sugar, minerals, fiber, fruits and vegetables moisten and loosen the stools. Too much, including milk, ice cream and cold drinks dilute, weaken and slow digestion and elimination (loose stools, diarrhea and constipation). Plant fiber, cellulose naturally absorbs, swells with water giving the stools bulk and form. Processed grains and starchy vegetables paste the stools increase the amount of toilet paper.

For simple cases of diarrhea, carob powder (2 tsp three to four times per day) and raspberry leaf tea are recommended in addition to the middle diet, adjusted accordingly. The initial, corrective diet should be light: toast and or tea (peppermint or cinnamon, both anti-diarrheas.). If it does not cease within a day or two, then contact a doctor, as diarrhea can also indicate **bacterial contamination**. Spices increase digestion, drain excess water while countering killing obnoxious bacteria, fungi, etc. Do not take magnesium when experiencing diarrhea as magnesium naturally softens the stools.

Diuretics

Diuretics help eliminate excess fluids (edema) via the production and secretion of urine. They also treat hypertension (high blood pressure) and congestive heart failure. Fruits, vegetables, spices and bitter herbs are diuretic in nature. Too many diuretics, bitter herbs, juices, cold drinks increase water retention and dryness. Cooked foods also increase urination.

The following herbs are natural **diuretics**:
- Horsetail, corn silk, coriander, parsley, poria
- Uva ursi, watercress, and watermelon seeds

Spices (heating, drying) increase urination and perspiration. Too many tend to dry and slow the urine. Diuretics increase the urge to urinate. Take during the day. Check with your doctor first. Smoking increases water retention.

Soft dairy (milk, yogurt, cottage cheese and ice cream), salads, juices and cold drinks in excess dilute, weaken and cool the digestion and elimination, causing excess, profuse urination.

Too much water, eight glasses per day, in the extreme, tends to weaken the kidneys and urinary bladder, causing more water to be retained (edema) than eliminated. Too much water can also weaken, cool digestive fire causing excess urination.

Dizziness

The brain is a function of blood, nutrients. Any sudden interruption or extreme reduction in blood flow to the brain (blood rich) via **blood deficiency** (via long-term low protein, low fat and high carbohydrate (salads, juices, cold drinks) diets), **clogged arteries** (via long-term high protein, high fat diets) or injury tends to impair, reduce mental function, awareness causing dizziness and in the extreme, unconsciousness. Alcohol, drugs, smoking, caffeine in the extreme, can also restrict blood flow, cause dizziness.

Protein and fat build, fuel all structure function. Too little thins and weakens the blood, and in the extreme, weakens decreases all function, mental and physical, causing a lack of holding, swaying and dizziness.

Thick blood (clots, high cholesterol) and clogged arteries (clogged) in the extreme, reduces circulation, blood flow to the head (dizziness, forgetfulness etc.), as does smoking, alcohol, caffeine, hot spices, animal and fried foods, which heat, dry, contract blood vessels, reducing their size, diameter, blood flow.

Dizziness is generally a stage 5 symptom, disease. The middle diet, adjusted accordingly is recommended. Avoid caffeine, alcohol, smoking, late night eating, processed grains, fried foods, etc. Medical consultation may also be necessary.

Dysmenorrhea

Dysmenorrhea is **painful menstruation**

- Intestinal cramps, bloating
- Nausea, vomiting
- Blood clots, excessive menstrual flow

High protein, high fat diets, overeating and alcohol tend to thicken the blood, which in turn, thickens clogs and weakens the liver. All blood passes through the liver.

The liver stores, cleanses (removes excess protein and fat) and releases the blood. High protein, high fat diets, especially animal, in the extreme, clog, thicken and weaken the liver. Less protein, fat and cholesterol are removed, more stays, thickens the blood (clots, high cholesterol) that eventually pass unevenly into the uterus, disrupting, distorting menstrual flow: pain, excessive bleeding, blood clots, dysmenorrhea, uterine tumors, endometriosis and or pelvic inflammatory disease. Obesity, uterine tumors, endometriosis (page 216) and or deficiency can also be a cause.

The colder middle diet is recommended for "hot", high protein, high fat dysmenorrhea.

- Eat less animal and grain (especially prior to the period) and more fruit, vegetables and spices.

- Bitter herbs (aloe vera, valerian, gotu kola, skullcap, myrrh, etc.) help move the blood.

- Spices (turmeric, cumin, coriander, fennel, etc.), help thin, move the blood, relax and unclog the liver.

The hotter middle diet is recommended for deficiency. Medical consultation, treatment may also be necessary. Dysmenorrhea takes months and or years to develop and consequently months and or years to cure, depending on severity, and or ability to discipline oneself.

Dysmenorrhea

- Stage 1: **Dietary cause**: long-term high protein, fat and starch diets, overeating, alcohol, tobacco
- Stage 2: **Digestion**: abdominal bloating, gas
- Stage 3: **Elimination**: constipation
- Stage 4: **Blood**: clots, high cholesterol
- Stage 5: **Circulation**: clogged arteries, menstrual clots, menstrual, intestinal cramps, pain, excessive menstruation, bleeding
- Stage 6: **Organs**: pelvic inflammatory disease, uterine tumors, endometriosis

19

"E- F" Diseases

Ear Infections

There are two types of ear infection, inflammation (otitis): external and internal.

- **External otitis**, infection of the outer ear can be caused by cosmetics, piercing or bacterial infection.

- **Internal otitis** of the inner ear (vertigo, loss of balance) and **otitis media** (affects the middle ear, behind eardrum) common in infants and children tends to be caused by extreme cold, damp diet, climate (winter, air conditioning, etc.), bacterial and or upper respiratory infections.

The **Eustachian tube** connects the **naso-pharynx** (nose, throat), middle ear and auditory tubes (connect the ear to the back of the nasal cavity). It regulates air pressure, temperature and moisture. **Excess moisture**, fluids can pass from the nose and throat into the ears (via the Eustachian tube), collect, stagnate, fester and infect with bacteria

- Inflame and pressurize the ear
- Earache, sharp, dull or throbbing pain
- Feeling of fullness in the ear, high fever

Low pressure, colder temperatures (winter, air conditioning, sleeping in cold, damp basement, etc.) tend to increase moisture in the lungs, throat, nose, etc.

Colder body temperatures (via diet or climate) harden fluids in the lungs, throat, nose and sinuses into excess water, mucous and or phlegm, which can pass and stagnate in the ears. Bacteria, viruses thrive in stagnant, watery mediums (mucous, urine) before inflaming, infecting.

Excess fluid→ Bacteria, virus→ infection→ inflammation

Middle ear infections are common in children (under developed) who tend to be cold, weak and damp, especially when they eat cold, damp diets (milk and cereal) or live in cold, damp climates (making them more susceptible to cold, damp diseases). High altitudes and colder temperatures increase discomfort and infection.

Protein, fat, cooked foods and digestion (three meals per day) heats and dries (regulates moisture) the body. Long-term cold, damp diets (milk, yogurt, soft cheese, ice cream, fruits, juices, sugar and cold drinks) tend to dilute and weaken digestion, which weakens cools and dampens the body.

Digestion transforms food into blood (nutrients energize and heat the body). Digestion (fiery process), three meals per day also heats and dries the body, especially the lungs, throat, sinuses, ears, which lie above the digestive organs. Heat rises. Too many salads, tropical fruits, juices, smoothies, cold drinks (includes ice water), sodas, etc. dilute, cool and decrease digestion (abdominal bloating, gas), elimination (loose stools) and nutrient absorption, blood, energy, body temperature. Weak digestion, deficient, low protein, fat blood also weakens the immune system, increasing the tendency to catch colds. Blood fuels immunity. The hotter middle diet (spices, cooking) is recommended, in addition to medical consultation and or treatment.

Spices increase digestion and dry dampness: mucous, phlegm, loose stools, edema, etc. Carrots, yams, apples can be used in baking (cookies) in place of sweeteners, to reduce sugar cravings. Cooked foods, soups, stew and spices (ginger, cinnamon used in cookies) heat the body. Hot cereals, nuts, seeds and spices are more warming, building than milk and cereal (cold, damp)

Garlic or peppermint oil drops in the ear dry dampness while fighting infection. Ear cones, candles and mullein, also dry excess fluids. The candles (different types) are placed in the ear and set on fire. As the cone, candle burns down, it absorbs water, dries the ear. Ear candles, made with wax may drip excess wax into the ears. Consult with a doctor first.

Eczema

Eczema, also known as atopic dermatitis is an inflammatory, red itchy condition of the skin that produces **blister like formations that weep**, release fluid before forming a crust, scale and or flake. Eczema in Chinese medicine and Ayurveda is defined as a cold, damp, kapha disease caused by deficiency of protein, fat, cooked foods, etc. and or too many sweets, sugar. Low levels of hydrochloric acid, Candidiasis or food allergies (possible dietary causes) are also a cause.

The skin builds up and breaks down (cleanses) largely according to diet. Too little building or too much cleansing, in the extreme, tends to

- Thins cracks, bleeds, infects and weeps (pus) the skin (eczema) on the hands, fingers, arms, knees

- Itching, scratching, scabs, etc.

The symptoms of eczema indicate **chronic deficiency** as the skin, more or less, is falling apart.

Protein and fat build, thicken, fuel and hold. Long-term cold, damp low protein, low fat (soft dairy) diets thin the blood. Long-term thin, low protein, low fat blood (deficiency) weakens thins the skin (eczema), hair, nails bones, organs, etc. Too many salads, tropical fruits, juices, cold drinks and sugar dilute, weaken digestion reducing nutrient absorption, blood.

Case history: In 1989, while living in Florida, I developed a bad, hideous case of eczema. It first started as a pimple, blister on my index finger (left hand) that quickly multiplied over the next few months into a multitude of blisters, cracked skin, bleeding, pus, covering all fingers, the entire back of my hand slowly moving up the back of the arm. Two fingers on my right hand were also starting to infect. This happened while I was running my health food store and going to acupuncture school. It was gross. I wore surgical gloves during the day. I tried every Chinese herbal remedy. Nothing worked. I eventually turned to Ayurvedic Medicine via **Ayurvedic Healing** by Dr. David Frawley, O.M.D., and **Yoga of Herbs** by Dr. Frawley and Dr. Vasant Lad, who recommended dietary changes and the use of spices (6+ per meal). My diet was bland, low protein, fat (soft dairy) and sweet, cold (grains, raw vegetables, tropical fruits, juices and cold drinks).

I increased protein, fat, cooked foods and spices (cumin, fennel, turmeric, cayenne. ginger, etc.), burdock tea, while reducing yogurt, salads, tropical and citrus fruits, juices, cold drinks, soda, etc. Within three weeks, my eczema cleared up. My digestion also got better: less bloating, gas, burping, farting, etc. I did have eczema as a teenager (not as serious).

Eczema and acne are not the same disease, as acne tends to be hot, inflammatory symptom, disease, caused by too much animal protein, fat, oil (salad dressings, cookies, candy, chips and chocolate) and sugar. The body converts all excess sugar into fat.

High protein, fat and starch diets, in the extreme, tend to cause hard, fixed, overbuilt symptoms: acne, warts, tumors, psoriasis, etc.

Cold, damp low protein and low fat diets, in the extreme, tend to cause eczema. The hotter middle diet is recommended.

Edema

Edema is the **accumulation of fluid** in the soft tissues and can occur anywhere in the body: head, arms, legs, etc. It is generally a cold, damp (kapha) disease, caused by poor diet, chronically weak digestion, drugs and or injury. Edema tends to attack **women** more than men, as many women tend to eat cold, damp diets soft dairy, fruits, juices, sugar). Men (testosterone, hot, building hormone, higher metabolism) tend to eat the opposite: high protein, high fat.

Body temperature (98.6°F) and digestion heats, protects and dries the body. Protein, fat build, fuel heat all structure, function. Too many cold, damp foods (milk, yogurt, cottage cheese, ice cream, citrus and tropical fruits, juices, smoothies, cold drinks, etc.) cools, dampens with excess fluids that overwhelm the lungs, kidneys and urinary bladder, which control perspiration and urination. Less fluid via perspiration and urination is eliminated, and more retained in the lungs, abdomen, thighs, ankles, arms, etc.

Too many cold drinks, especially ice water with meals, dilute and weaken digestion, which is the ultimate fat, water and sugar burner. Digestion, three meals per day heat and dry the body, eliminate excess fluids perspiration, defecation and urination.

Overwork lack of sleep, excessive sex, drugs also drain, and weaken the kidneys and urinary bladder.

The hotter middle diet, spices (for cold, damp diseases) is recommended. Reduce animal food, nuts, oils, salads; tropical fruits, juices, sodas, cold drinks, ice cream, late dinners and late night eating, which can weaken digestion, metabolism. **Spices** in vegetable soups, stews strengthen digestion, drain excess fluids. **Diuretics** help eliminate excess water as does exercise

- Alfalfa, burdock, corn silk, parsley
- Horsetail, juniper berry

Endometriosis

Endometriosis is the abnormal presence, excessive growth (hot) of endometrial cells, tissues (outside its normal location in the uterine lining) in the uterine walls, fallopian tubes, ovaries and or bowels,) It tends to cause

- Dysmenorrhea, painful menses, pain in uterus and lower back, excessive bleeding before the period, blood clots
- Nausea, vomiting, constipation
- Dysuria (painful urination), painful sex

Too much protein, fat especially animal and fried foods thicken the blood (stagnant blood), endometrial tissue too much, causing inflammation, disease.

The colder middle diet, meal plan, bitter herbs (turmeric, golden seal, myrrh, etc.) is recommended. Reduce animal protein, fat, oily foods, overeating and late meals. Eat more raw fruit and vegetables, beans, etc.

Eyes

The eyes receive light through the **pupil** (opens and closes) and **lens** that adjust, refract light images directly on the **retina** (connects to the **optic nerve**, brain). Blood, nutrients build, fuel, stimulate, moisten the eyes, lens, optic nerve, brain, etc. Less blood, nutrients dry weaken. **Protein and fat** build thicken, moisten and fuel. Water, minerals, etc. thin, cool.

.
- **Long-term blood deficiency** via long-term low protein, low fat and high carbohydrate (fruits, juices, sugar, cold drinks) diets, thin the blood, decrease circulation, especially to the extremities: head, arms and legs.

- **Too much protein and fat** tends to thicken and clog the **blood** (clots, high cholesterol) and **arteries** (plaque, atherosclerosis) reducing circulation, blood, nutrients especially to the extremities.

- Too much protein, fat also tends to cause **bumps**, growths on the **eyelids**.

- Overeating and clogged intestines concentrate blood in the abdomen; reduce blood flow to the head.

- Too much reading, television can also weaken the eyes.

Case history: My vision started going bad at age 53. I had to buy magnifying glasses to read paperback novels. At age 54, I added *organic* **carrot tops** to my diet (middle). After a few months of eating cooked organic carrot tops (in vegetable soups) in addition to less animal protein, fat, my vision restored to 20:20. I no longer read with glasses. I also rarely drink coffee, do not smoke and have been eating the middle diet for many years giving me a greater, faster healing ability.

Horsetail, bilberry, Ginkgo Biloba and Eye-bright increase circulation of blood to the brain and are commonly used to improve vision. There are also exercises to strengthen the eyes muscles (that hold the lens). The "Bates Method" is one set of exercises. Avoid, reduce caffeine, smoking and alcohol. Check with your doctor.

Fear

It takes energy, strength to be courageous. Chronic blood, protein, fat and jing deficiency tends to cause fear (of falling down, breaking bones easily), which is generally associated with the kidneys (store jing) and old age. Jing (sexual essence) is the fundamental substance of the marrow, bones. It naturally declines with age, use.

Young people do not fear bone breaks, as their bones (jing+) heal quickly. They exhibit more bravery and less fear, unlike children (underdeveloped, less jing) and the elderly (less energy, jing). On a spiritual level, fear shows a lack of faith in God, as there is nothing to fear. The middle diet, adjusted accordingly and reduction of sex is recommended.

Fever

Normal body temperature is approximately 98.6°F and runs slightly higher during the day, and in women, especially after ovulation. A fever is an elevation in body temperature. The body generally raises its temperature produces a fever to burn eliminate excess cold (common cold), bacteria, viruses, etc. Sweating, hot soups, spicy foods, alcohol, hot baths and bacterial infections also raise body temperature produce a fever. Severe fevers, higher body temperatures require medical attention. Fevers in general are a good thing (healthy), but not good when excessive.

Fibrocystic breasts

Fibrocystic breasts are a non-cancerous condition characterized by soft, freely moving **cysts** (closed fluid filled sac) or lumps in the breast, generally caused by poor diet and monthly changes in hormonal levels (estrogen, progesterone). Cysts tend to be cold, damp.

Body temperature (98.6°F) and digestion (three meals a day), heats and dries (maintains, thins fluids) the body, especially the lungs, breasts (heat rises, moves up and out).

Long-term cold, damp diet (milk, yogurt, soft cheese, ice cream, tropical fruits, juices, smoothies, shakes, cold drinks and sugar) dilute, cool and weaken digestion, decrease nutrient absorption, blood, energy, heat, body temperature.

Colder, lower body temperatures harden fluids in the chest, lungs, breasts, uterus, etc. into mucous, phlegm, cysts, etc.

The hotter middle diet (less animal, nuts and oil) is recommended. Spices, cooked foods, help eliminate excess water. Regular examination (personally and professionally) of the breasts is advisable

Fibroids, uterine

Uterine fibroids are benign (harmless) growths that form on the interior muscular wall and or exterior of the uterus. They usually form during the late thirties and or early forties, and then disappear after menopause suggesting a causal relationship with estrogen (growth hormone). Estrogen supplements and high protein, high fat diets, in the extreme, build, stimulate excessive growth, tissue (tumors, fibroids). The colder middle diet is and medical consultation is recommended.

Fibromyalgia

Fibromyalgia Syndrome (FMS) is a rheumatic disorder, autoimmune disease that tends to attack women more so than men. The general cause is poor diet. The following symptoms characterize FMS:

- Chronic, achy muscular pain, extreme fatigue
- Dizziness, loss of balance
- Impaired coordination, stiffness in the morning
- Chemical or food allergies
- Constipation, diarrhea, Irritable Bowel Syndrome
- Insomnia, memory loss, headaches

FMS tends to attack women beginning in young adulthood. This is due in large part to anemic diet and menstruation (blood loss). Anemic, low protein, low fat diets and blood loss weaken digestion elimination, nutrient absorption, blood, circulation, etc.

The symptoms, pain of Fibromyalgia, similar to most autoimmune diseases (pages 172- 4) indicate chronic cold, deficiency, stage 5+ disease.

All diseases progress in stages. **Poor diet**: Long-term cold, damp low protein, low fat (soft dairy) and high carbohydrate (bread, salads, tropical fruits, juices, sugar, etc.) diets tend to dilute, weaken and slow

- **Digestion** (abdominal bloating, gas)
- **Elimination** (loose stools, constipation)
- **Nutrient absorption, blood** (blood deficiency)
- **Circulation** (reduced)

Deficient, thin blood tends to reduce circulation, especially to the extremities causing

- Fatigue, pain, pallor, coldness
- Dry, thin and or cracked skin
- Inflammation of the joints, dryness, stiffness
- Dizziness, loss of balance, impaired coordination
- Memory loss, insomnia, amenorrhea, PMS

The hotter middle diet for cold, deficiency is recommended.

Forgetfulness

The brain, memory functions according to its blood, nutrients supply, especially protein and fat (build, fuel). Blood deficiency (via low protein, low fat diets) and or decreased circulation via clogged, narrow arteries (via high protein, high fat diets, smoking, etc.) starves the brain, nerves, causing forgetfulness (lack of holding, deficiency). The middle diet, meal plan, adjusted accordingly is recommended.

Frigidity

Frigidity is characterized by a general lack of sexual desire and or inability to orgasm. It is generally associated with women more so than men (testosterone, hot). Frigidity has both physiological and psychological causes including sexual trauma during childhood, adolescence, anxiety, depression, insufficient lubrication, inadequate stimulation, anemia, poor diet and or chronic illness.

Diet is one factor as life, sex require fuel, protein and fat. You cannot have a fire (sexual energy, desire, orgasm) without fuel. Low protein, low fat and high carbohydrate diets tend to reduce, cool all energy, including sexual. Many women tend to eat cold, damp, low protein, low fat (milk, yogurt, ice cream, beans, etc.) and high carbohydrate (salads, fruits, juices) diets. The hotter middle diet is advised, if coldness, anemic diet is the cause.

20

"G- H" Diseases

Gallstones

The gall bladder is a pear shaped, organ 3-4" in size, located on right side of the body, connected to the liver and small intestine. The liver stores, cleanses (removes cholesterol, poisons, toxins, etc.) and releases the blood. Poisons, toxins are transformed into bile, cholesterol, lecithin and other substances. Bile emulsifies, digests fat. One pint of bile per day passes into the gall bladder and is released into the small intestine (via cystic and bile ducts). Unused bile moves down into the large intestine, mixed and eliminated with the feces.

Abnormal concentration of **bile acids, cholesterol** (byproduct of protein and fat digestion) and **phospholipids** (in the bile) tend to create stones (cholelithiasis) in the gall bladder.

Gallstones can move into the ducts and cause nausea, vomiting and or pain in the right side, upper abdomen. They can also inflame the gall bladder (cholecystitis) cause nausea, fever and pain in abdomen or behind the breastbone. The urine may become tea or coffee colored. Symptoms tend to occur after a fried or fatty meal. Gall bladder attacks mimic the pain of heart attack.

75% of all gallstones are **cholesterol stones**. High animal protein, saturated fat (high in cholesterol), sugar and alcohol, in the extreme, tend to cause stones in the gall bladder and kidneys. All excess sugar turns into fat.

The colder middle diet spices (fennel, cumin and coriander), bitter and diuretic herbs (aloe vera, horsetail, burdock, corn silk, uva ursi, and catnip) to reduce, digest and eliminate excess fat, cholesterol and stones is recommended.

Folk remedy: drink 1tsp each of **apple cider vinegar and honey** in a glass of apple juice, water several times during the day, and or drink three TB's **olive oil in lemon juice** right before bedtime, lie; sleep on your right side; for 1-2 nights to help eliminate gallstones. Rhubarb and cascara sagrada may also help. Check with your doctor and research further before using.

GIRD and GERD

Gastrointestinal Reflux Disorder (GIRD) and Gastro Esophageal Reflux Disease (GERD) are two common digestive disorders that share similar symptoms:

- Abdominal bloating, gas, nausea
- Acidic or sour taste in the mouth, throat
- Heartburn, burning sensation and or pain in the stomach, chest or behind the breastbone
- Shortness of breath

Poor diet, too much protein, fat and starch or too little protein, fat and cleansing (fruits, vegetables) tends to cause poor digestion, GIRD, GERD. The **stomach** is the first digestive organ to receive, process food, which it mixes with hydrochloric acid (HCl) and other enzymes specifically designed to digest animal protein, fat. This mixture sits, **ferments** (souring process) and dissolves, before moving down into the small intestine, for further digestion, nutrient absorption. Whatever food, fluids not digested, absorbed, become waste.

The throat, stomach and small intestine are more or less one long tube (30+ feet) that connects to another long tube, large intestine (5 feet) ending in the anus.

Overeating, especially protein, fat and starch (bread, cookies, etc.) increase the production of HCl while also obstructing and slowing the downward movement of food, causing it to collect, stagnate (**bloating**), ferment (**sour**) and eventually back up, rebel: **burping, sour breath, heartburn, nausea, vomiting**, etc. like a clogged pipe that overflows. Obesity, tight clothing and pregnancy also tend to obstruct the downward movement of food, causing a back flow of HCl, heartburn.

The pain, burning of heartburn is caused by the backflow of hydrochloric acid (HCl) into the esophagus. HCl in the extreme irritates and burns sensitive tissues. Esophageal sphincter muscles that control the opening and closing of the valve that connects the esophagus to the stomach generally prevent its back flow.

- Long-term low protein, low fat diets tend to weaken, slow digestion, movement of food.
- Too many juices, cold drinks dilute and weaken digestive acid and enzymes, slow the movement of food (abdominal bloating, gas, burping).
- Too many processed grains (bread, noodles, cookies, chips, etc.) paste, narrow and or clog the stomach and intestines (heartburn, burning sensation, pasty stools).

The middle diet, meal plan, adjusted accordingly is recommended. Spices, Kim Chi (Korean spicy cabbage), raw celery and lettuce (help reduce heartburn), and walking help move food stagnation and or relieve heartburn. Reduce grains, salads, tropical fruits, cold drinks, soft dairy, etc.

Case history: A female customer of mine was having digestive problems. Every time she ate, she would experience abdominal bloating, gas, burping, pain and heartburn. Her diet was anemic: low protein, low fat and high carbohydrate (pasta, bread, salads, fruit, juices, etc.). I suggested **fennel seeds** (1/4 tsp after each meal) in addition to the **hotter, middle diet.**

Three weeks later, she came back and hugged me. Her digestive problems, constipation and hot flashes (which she had not told me about) had disappeared. I asked her age. She was 43 years old. I told her that her hot flashes were not caused by menopause but instead by intestinal heat via indigestion, **stagnation** of food, waste. Her doctor had diagnosed her as menopausal; which I thought was a little premature. Stagnation of energy, food, etc. tends to generate heat.

Gout

Gout is a common type of arthritis that tends to attack men, more so than women. It is caused by **excess uric acid** (sodium urate) in the blood that crystallizes into needle shaped deposits in the tissues jabbing, paining and inflaming the bones, joints, especially the **big toe**. Uric acid is a byproduct of protein digestion, especially animal and fried foods.

Too much protein tends to cause excess uric acid, crystals, pain, inflammation, arthritis.

Too little, in the extreme, decreases the production of urinase (digestive enzyme makes uric acid water-soluble), which tends to cause excess uric acid in the blood. Heredity and chronic illness can also be a factor, but the major cause is diet.

Many men tend to eat a "rich" high protein, high fat diet, unlike women, who tend to eat the opposite: low protein, low fat. Many men tend to develop high protein, high fat symptoms: clots, high cholesterol, atherosclerosis, high blood pressure, gout, arthritis, warts, tumors, kidney and gallstones, cancer, etc.

The colder middle diet (less beans, nuts, and yogurt) is recommended. Eat less, space and or skip meals. Overeating clogs the liver. Drink water between meals. Eat fruit as a dessert. Dinner is always the smallest meal. Reduce nighttime eating. Bitter herbs (golden seal, aloe vera, turmeric) dissolve fat and help cleanse the blood Check with your doctor first.

Gums (bleeding)

Poor diet (overeating, especially protein, fat, oil, flour and sweets), poor dental hygiene and or smoking tends to cause the gums to bleed and or recede. The middle diet, meal plan is recommended, in addition to flossing, Xylitol toothpaste, raspberry leaf tea, peppermint oil (page 281), barberry root and regular cleanings to keep gums clean. More info (page 282)

Hair Loss

Hair is a living tissue, follicle, nourished primarily by protein, fat and jing, which build, fuel all structure function. It is natural for the hair to thin and lose its color as one gets older, starting around age forty. Poor diet and excessive sex accelerate hair loss. Genetics, heredity is also a factor as some people are genetically predisposed towards baldness. Others eat poorly or sexually exhaust themselves accelerating their loss of hair.

High protein, fat diets, in the extreme, tend to cause high cholesterol, atherosclerosis (clogged, narrow arteries), which reduces, circulation, blood, flow to the head: fatigue, pallor, memory loss, hair loss (crown, top, center of head), etc. Overeating, especially protein, fat, oil and starch tends to dry the scalp, hair and create white flakes, dandruff (excess shedding of skin).

Low protein, low fat diets, in the extreme, thin the blood (blood deficiency), which eventually thins the hair (especially in the front), skin, nails, bones, etc. It is the major reason why hair loss is becoming more common among women (low protein, low fat diets).

Hair is also made from **jing** (sexual essence, ovum, sperm, etc.). The bones, hair, memory, etc. are strong, full when jing is full (fountain of youth) and weak, thin and dry when declining (starts after sexual maturation). Excessive, daily sex (masturbation, orgasm) especially in men drains jing; accelerates the aging, drying process, as does the daily consumption of coffee (caffeine is the worst), tobacco and alcohol. Taoist medicine advises men to restrict, forgo the ejaculation, orgasm and or sex (celibacy) to retain, conserve jing, to slow aging, drying, hair loss, etc.

Proper diet, herbs and conservation of jing improve the skin, hair, bones, skin, memory, etc. The middle diet, meal plan, adjusted accordingly is recommended. **Black sesame seeds** (organic, ground, nut and seed mill), black fungus and black beans nourish hair, jing and the kidneys. Fenugreek seeds, **brewers yeast, lecithin, niacin, biotin and Fo ti** promote the growth of hair. Sage tea as a hair wash also helps. Avoid overeating, alcohol, smoking, caffeine, refined sugar and excessive use of bitter herbs.

Hearing Loss

There are three categories of hearing loss. **Conductive** hearing loss occurs when the ear canal is blocked (earwax), infected, inflamed and or damaged. **Sensor neural** hearing loss is damage to the inner ear and or nerves (acoustical) via birth, prescription medications, antibiotics, non-steroidal anti-inflammatory drugs, viral infections, etc. It starts as an inability to hear high pitch sounds before progressing to lower pitched sounds and **neural** hearing loss caused by brain tumor or stroke.

The mechanics of hearing: Sound waves enter the outer ear and vibrate the **eardrum** (tympanic membrane), bones of the middle ear and **hair cells** in the inner ear. The vibrations are transmitted to the brain via the **auditory nerve**.

The loss of hearing occurs when passage of sound waves to the brain is blocked via

- Excessive earwax, infection, loud noises
- Changes in atmospheric pressure, trauma
- Bathing and or swimming in contaminated water
- Poor circulation

The brain, ear and auditory nerve are also a function of blood, nutrients (building and cleansing). Diet, herbs can improve hearing loss, depending on severity. Check with your doctor get an examination, as diet may not be the cause.

Protein and fat build, fuel. Long-term low protein, low fat and high carbohydrate diets weaken, decrease all structure and function, including hearing.

Too much protein and fat, in the extreme, thickens, clogs the blood and arteries reducing blood flow, especially to the head. Less blood, nutrients produces less function, hearing loss, poor vision, etc.

Extreme cold, damp weather or diet can also adversely affect the ear. The **middle ear** is connected to the **nasopharynx** (region of throat behind the ear) via the **Eustachian tube**. The throat is connected to the lungs. Internal and external cold and damp (air, water) can penetrate the body, attack the lungs and pass directly into ears via the throat and Eustachian tube. Cold air hardens and stagnate fluids in the ears, which can disrupt, weaken hearing and or cause earaches and middle ear infections.

Body temperature (98.6°F) and digestion (three meals per day) heats and dries the body. Lower body temperatures cool and harden body fluids in the same way colder temperatures harden water in the air into rain, snow and ice. In the body colder temperatures via long-term blood, protein and fat deficiency, chronically weak digestion or age (children, under developed and the elderly, less energy) cools, hardens and stagnates water in the lungs, throat, ears, sinuses, nose, etc.

Too many cold, damp foods and drinks (milk, ice cream, salads, juices, sodas and cold drinks) dilute, weaken digestive fire, which in turn decreases nutrient absorption, blood, energy, heat, body temperature.

Most bacterial and viral infections require a fluid medium to grow. Trapped water in the ears provides an excellent opportunity, medium for growth. Spicy herbs: **garlic or peppermint oil** drops in the ear dry dampness, which in turn, fights, destroys infection.

Ear candles also help. They are placed in the ear and the tip is set on fire. As the cone, candle burns down, it absorbs water, dries the ear. There are different types of ear candles. Ear candles, made with wax may drip wax into the ears.

One-third of all people over age 65 have hearing problems via **reduced blood supply** to ear via

- Heart disease, diabetes, clogged arteries
- Poor diet

Tinnitus (constant or recurring loud or soft ringing, buzzing in the ears) may also occur. **Loud** ringing generally indicates overbuilt, high protein, high fat conditions: liver congestion, high cholesterol, atherosclerosis, high blood pressure etc. **Low** ringing, pitch indicates weakness, deficiency: anemia, low blood pressure and is generally associated with the kidneys.

Middle ear infections are common in children. Children tend to be weak, cold as they are underdeveloped, still developing. This weakness, lack of energy, heat makes them more susceptible to cold, damp, especially if eating a cold, damp diet (milk and cereal, juices, cold drinks, sugar, etc.).

The hotter middle diet, meal plan for cold, damp is recommended. Cooked foods, soups, stews, beans, warm and dry the body, lungs, throat, ears, nose, etc. Spices increase digestion and dry dampness: mucous, phlegm, loose stools, edema, cellulite, etc.

Ginger and cinnamon in cookies, spices in soup, are an easy, tasty delivery system. Reduce all cold foods. Milk and cereal (cold, damp) is more of a dessert than a breakfast, and should be avoided.

The following are symptoms of hearing deficit in **infants, children**:

- Failure to blink or react to loud noises
- Sleeps through loud noises
- Failure to turn head toward familiar sounds
- Mono-tonal babbling
- Failure to speak clearly by age two
- No interest in word games or being read to
- Habitual yelling or screaming when communicating
- Shyness, withdrawal

Hearing deficit is more severe, sometimes caused by genetics. It requires a thorough medical examination.

Hepatitis, A, B and C

Hepatitis is inflammation of the liver. It is generally caused by viral infection. The liver filters harmful substances: toxins, dead cells, fats, hormones, bilirubin (yellow pigment of bile), etc. from the blood. The following are general symptoms of hepatitis: abdominal pain, fever, nausea, vomiting, dark urine, light-colored stools, loss of appetite, weakness, headaches, muscle aches, joint pains, drowsiness and or jaundice (yellowing of skin). Poor diet (high protein, high fat, alcohol, sugar) can also weaken, infect, inflame and enlarge the liver.

There are three main viruses (hepatitis).

- **Hepatitis A** is infectious hepatitis, easily spread via contaminated foods, water, etc.

- **Hepatitis B** is serum hepatitis, easily spread via blood transfusions, contaminated needles, etc. Most recover. Twenty-five per cent develops into cirrhosis or liver cancer.

- **Hepatitis C** contracted via blood transfusions, needles, sex is the most serious.

Too much protein, fat, especially animal, fried foods, alcohol and overeating in the extreme, tends to clog, weaken and inflame the liver providing the future breeding ground for Hepatitis.

The middle diet, meal plan, adjusted accordingly and medical treatment is recommended. Reduce all saturated fat: red meat, chicken, pizza, fries, chips, oils, etc. Turkey once a day is permitted. Increase nuts and seeds (helps break down excess fat, cholesterol), vegetables, cooked and raw (3-5): Reduce tropical fruits, juices, salads, cooked tomatoes, potatoes, tobacco, alcohol and drugs. Eat small amounts of fruit. Avoid overeating, eat less, skip or space the meals.

Spices increase digestion, burn, metabolize excess fat (cholesterol), water (mucous, phlegm), bacteria, viruses, and help purify the blood.

Green tea and **chrysanthemum tea** also aid, increase digestion, elimination of excess fat.

Bitter herbs (golden seal, gentian) help eliminate noxious bacteria, viruses but *contraindicated* when there is dampness (edema, loose stools, etc) or weak digestion.

Enzymatic Therapy and other vitamin companies make specific formulas for hepatitis (more info: **Prescription for Nutritional Healing.** Eat well as poor diet will undermine any supplement, drug.

Some herbs, spices may conflict with prescription drugs. Medical consultation and or treatment may be necessary.

Herpes

Herpes is a group of viruses that cause painful blister-like skin eruptions. In TCM, herpes is defined, caused by a combination of **wind** (spreads fast, easily), **heat** (raised, red eruptions) and **damp** (oozing sores).

The colder middle diet, meal plan, **bitter herbs** (gentian, sarsaparilla) is recommended. Use light spices (fennel, cumin and coriander). Avoid, alcohol, tobacco, caffeine, red meat, pork, fried foods, sugary desserts, which accelerate, increase wind, heat and dampness. TCM, **acupuncture**, bleeds the eyes of the knees (look for dark capillaries) to possibly lessen and or cure herpes. Consult an Acupuncturist.

Case history one of my customers (woman) was able to reduce her attacks via diet (vegetables, fruits and low protein, low fat), herbs and acupuncture to one or two attacks per year. Everything, including viruses requires not only a host but also a dietary plan, support. Disease also has its own diet. Do not feed it. Beet green soup also helps (**Tao of Nutrition** by Maoshing Ni, p. 29).

Hiatus hernia

Hiatus hernia is a condition when part of the stomach protrudes through the diaphragm. Sometimes it causes no symptoms, other times acid reflux and heartburn. Overeating and obesity are general causes. Too much food, especially protein, fat and starch (noodles, bread, cookies, chips, etc.) bloats and or pastes the stomach, small and large intestine, causing them to press on and or protrude. The colder middle diet is recommended. Eat less. Consult with a medical doctor.

High blood pressure (hypertension)

Blood pressure is the force of blood on the walls of the arteries produced by the contraction of the heart. Normal blood pressure is approximately 120/80. Higher number indicate high blood pressure, caused in general by high protein, high fat diets. The colder middle diet, bitter herbs is recommended. More info: page 126, 176

Hot Flashes

Hot flashes are *temporary* flashes of heat generally associated with menopause. Menopause represents a dual decline in blood and jing. Blood and jing moisten and cool, while also restraining heat. Age, excessive sex, low protein, low fat diet and caffeine deplete jing and blood, which fails to contain, cool and moisten normal surges of energy (heat) resulting in temporary escape, flash of heat. Stagnant energy via clogged intestines, arteries, obesity also causes "sudden" hot flashes, which dissipate once the obstruction passes.

Hot flashes tend to indicate blood, protein and fat **deficiency** as the fire, flash is **temporary**, due to low fuel, which produces a shorter fire. High fuel (excess animal protein, fat, coffee, tobacco and alcohol) produces, sustains a longer lasting fire, higher body temperature, excessive perspiration, etc. Excess causes excess. Deficiency causes deficiency.

The colder middle diet for blood deficiency is recommended. **Sage tea, pear juice, peppermint tea** and **Progesterone cream** help counter hot flashes. I sold a lot or progesterone cream in my health food store (17 years) and heard only praise. Check with your doctor.

Hysteria

Hysteria (neurotic disorder generally associated with menopause) has mental and physical causes. Long-term jing, blood, protein and fat deficiency thins and weakens the hair, skin, nails, bones, nerves, brain, emotions, attention span, rationality, memory, etc. Menopause represents a dual decline in jing (hormone, estrogen) and blood. Long-term blood deficiency (via long-term low protein, low fat and high carbohydrate diet) is a major factor that can predispose one (male or female) to hysteria. Hysteria is a deficiency symptom. It shows a lack of control via mental degeneration, poor circulation, blood deficiency, clogged arteries, poor diet, etc.

Many women tend to eat low protein, low fat diets and drink coffee, which are why hysteria is now attacking more and more women, especially at younger ages. Low protein and low fat diets do not adequately replace blood lost during menstruation causing an overall blood and chi deficiency, which not only attacks the reproductive organs but also the brain, nerves, emotions, etc. causing weakened, hysterical responses.

Blood, protein and fat deficiency can also attack men. It just takes a longer time to manifest, which is why men generally do not show the adverse effects of low protein, low fat diets, as quickly. The hotter middle diet, meal plan is recommended. Avoid red meat, veal, pork, etc. Eat (do not overeat) more eggs, chicken, turkey, hard cheese, etc. in addition to vegetables and fruit.

21

"I- J" Diseases

Infertility

Fertility is a function of nutrition. Protein and fat (especially animal) build, fuel the ovum, ovaries, uterus, fetus, pregnancy,   etc. Water, minerals, sugar, fruit, vegetables reduce, cleanse, cool. There are three dietary pathologies. More info: pregnancy (p. 263)

- Low protein, low fat diets and caffeine (reduces jing) thin the blood, ovum, ovaries, decrease fertility.

- Too many cold, damp foods, drinks, sugar reduces digestion, nutrient absorption, blood.

The hotter middle diet is recommended.

- High protein, fat diets, in the extreme tends to cause growths; tumors in the ovaries, uterus, and fallopian tubes (prevent the egg from descending into the uterus) that inhibit conception.

The colder middle diet, meal is recommended.

Inflammation

Blood (water, nutrients, etc.) moistens and cools the skin, muscles, tendons, ligaments, nerves, etc. Decreased blood flow to the tissues via long-term blood, protein and fat deficiency or clogged arteries **dry and inflame** the skin, muscles, tendons, nerves, etc.

Inflammation requires dryness via less blood (blood is moistening) to burn, inflame.

Long-term low protein, low fat diets weaken, thin the blood (blood deficiency), reduce circulation, especially to the extremities. Long-term high protein, high fat diets tend to clog and narrow the arteries, reduce blood flow, as does smoking, sedentary lifestyle, lack of exercise, etc. Regular exercise circulates the blood, moistens all the tissues. A moving gate gathers no rust. Injury (sprains) also cause inflammation via reduced blood flow.

Hot herbs (spices), internally (diet) and externally applied (salves) increase circulation of blood. Heat moves, spreads blood, moisture to the area that is dry, inflamed. The middle diet, adjusted accordingly, is recommended. Mullein helps nerve inflammation.

Insomnia

In TCM, the shen (spirit, consciousness) resides in the brain and heart (anchors the spirit). The heart and brain are blood, protein and fat rich. During the day (sun), the shen rises into the head, stimulating the brain, thinking. At night, it sinks down into the heart to sleep rejuvenate. Anything (food, television, reading, etc.) that heats, stimulates the body mind during the night stimulates thinking, dreaming, wakefulness, insomnia (inability to fall or stay asleep, or shallow, dream disturbed sleep).

Sleeping is a cooling (yin) activity, function that rejuvenates the body mind. It is difficult to fall asleep, stay sleep, no dreams, etc. when the body mind is overheated, cold or blood deficient. The need to sleep long hours decreases with age.

- The sun stimulates the body mind, which is why it is difficult to sleep during the day.

- Protein, fat, cooked foods, spices, alcohol, caffeine, smoking and overeating **heat** the body.

- Television, reading books and certain types (rock and roll, rap) of music stimulate, **heat** the mind.

- Blood deficiency fails to moisten, but instead **heats** (deficient heat) the body. It also weakens the heart's ability to store, anchor the shen (spirit)

- Jing, blood, milk, fruits, vegetables, juices, cold drinks, bitter herbs, resting, meditation and nighttime **cool, relax** the body.

There are two types of insomnia: acute and chronic.

- **Acute** (sudden) insomnia is relatively easy to cure via supplements, herbs (valerian), meditation, relaxation exercises etc., and reduction, elimination of acute, sudden causes (caffeine, spicy foods, late night television, reading, etc.).

- **Chronic** (long-term) insomnia is more difficult to cure as all chronic long-lasting diseases take months, years to not only develop but also cure.

Poor diet tends to cause insomnia.

(1) Long-term low protein, low fat diets tend to thin the blood (blood deficiency). Chronically thin blood thins, dries and weakens the heart, holding power, especially during the night allowing the sprit to rise up, into the head stimulating thinking, dreaming. The hotter middle diet is recommended.

(2) Too many cold, damp foods: milk, yogurt, ice cream, salads, fruits, juices, cold drinks (sodas, smoothies, ice water, etc.) cool, dampen the body, cause excess mucous, phlegm to form, collect in the nose, sinuses, throat and lungs which shortens, disrupts the breath (coughing, snoring) making it difficult to stay asleep (sleep apnea).

The hotter middle diet, spices (for cold, damp) is recommended. **Spices** dry fluids, mucous, etc., while also opening the sinuses, allowing the breath to flow freely, smoothly. Avoid spicy dinners (too hot, stimulating).

(3) Long-term high animal protein, fat, fried foods, diets, tend to thicken, harden, tense, dry and overheat the body making it difficult to physically relax, fall and stay sleep

- Protein and fat build thicken fuel and heat. Too much thickens the blood too much (clots, high cholesterol), which in turn thickens, clogs pastes and narrows the **arteries** with plaque (atherosclerosis), which in turn, raises blood pressure, body temperature.

- Protein, fat and starch (processed grains) thickens, pastes (insulates) the **small and large intestines** (polyps, bloating, gas, pain, constipation, etc.), skin, thighs, hips, etc. preventing the loss of heat, while increasing body temperature.

For severe "hot" insomnia, the colder middle diet: milk (dairy, non-dairy), 60% vegetables, raw and cooked, fruit, brewers yeast, biotin (before sleep), **bitter herbs** (1- 3 weeks), less eating, especially after 6:00 P.M., deep breathing and meditation are recommended.

Bitter herbs (laxative in nature) and less eating, especially protein, fat and starch drain excess heat, fat. Too much bitter weakens, dries the blood. Biotin (sublingual) before sleep helps cool, relax the body, heart, chest. Check with your doctor first.

Less protein, fat thins the blood. Raw fruit and vegetables (celery) make excellent nighttime snacks, although too much fruit may increase the urge to urinate. Chamomile teas, aloe vera juice, gel in juice 1- 2 times per day, also helps cool the body.

(4) Too much grain, especially processed (bread, cookies, etc.) tends to paste, harden and overheat the intestines. Clogged intestines tend to clog the nostrils making it difficult to breathe, sleep. The lungs (includes nose, sinuses, etc.) and large intestine are related, paired organs. Bitter herbs are.

Sleeping, lying on the right side generally opens the left nasal passage (more relaxing), unless you have liver congestion. Breathing through the right nostril is more stimulating.

(5) Caffeine, hot spices (dinner) and smoking overheats the body, tends to cause insomnia.

(6) Excessive sex drains jing, which in turn, fails to cool, moisten, but instead overheats (deficient) the body.

(7) Poor posture, misalignment, injury, excessive emotions, thoughts or environment disturbances (climate, electromagnetic radiation, noise, etc.) can also be a cause Regular exercise and proper diet (fruits, vegetables) dissipates excess heat, energy, which relaxes, cools the body.

Irritable Bowel Syndrome

Irritable Bowel Syndrome (IBS), also known as intestinal neurosis, mucous colitis and spastic colitis is a chronic digestive and eliminative disorder generally caused by long-term poor diet. It has the following symptoms:

- Abdominal bloating, pain, gas, nausea
- Mucous in the stools, constipation, diarrhea
- Colitis (inflammation of the colon), anorexia
- Tends to attack women, twice as much as men

The large intestine is largely a function of diet and digestion. Food, nutrients and non-nutrients (includes fiber) not digested, absorbed in the small intestine becomes waste that passes into the large intestine (cecum, **ascending, transverse and descending colon**, and rectum).

Long-term cold, damp diet (milk, yogurt, soft cheese, ice cream, grains, especially processed (bread, cookies, chips, etc.), salads, tropical fruits, juices, smoothies, cold drinks and sugar) diets tend to

- Dilute, weaken and slow **digestion** (abdominal bloating, pain, gas, nausea)

- Dilute, weaken and slow **elimination** (loose stools, mucous, constipation) while increasing waste, as all food, nutrients not digested, absorbed becomes waste transported to the large intestine. Excess waste pastes, clogs and inflames the colon (colitis).

- Decrease nutrient absorption, blood (anorexia)

- Many women tend to eat cold, damp diets.

The hotter middle diet for cold, deficient IBS is recommended.

Case history: One of my customers was suffering from IBS. Her daily, weekly symptoms were abdominal bloating, gas, loose stools, constipation, headaches and swelling (arms and legs swollen twice their size). I diagnosed her condition as a cold, damp, weak spleen (digestion). Her long-term diet was low protein, low fat and high carbohydrate (salads and juices). Her spleen, digestion became weak, cold producing the aforementioned symptoms. I recommended the hotter middle diet, cooked foods, spices, etc. in addition to a reduction in cold foods, drinks. **Week by week her condition got better.** Nine months later, most of her symptoms had disappeared, including the swelling in her arms and legs. She was very happy.

A year later, she went to see a nutritionist ($300) who took a stool sample, found excessive bacteria and recommended golden seal (cold, bitter herb), nine capsules a day. I had originally diagnosed coldness and deficiency as the cause of her condition, which she re-aggravated once she started taking golden seal. I explained to her why her symptoms had reappeared and refused to sell her golden seal.

Itching

Chronic itching, scratching is generally of symptom of excess energy, heat trapped in the liver, lungs, skin and or large intestine. The scratching, itching is an attempt to release heat via the puncturing, bleeding of the skin. Oily, fatty foods (meat, pork, chicken, chips, fries, nuts, etc.), spices, chocolate, coffee, alcohol and smoking overheat dry the body.

Smoking (tobacco, marijuana) is extremely heating, drying and toxic (poisons, heavy metals). The colder middle diet (less nuts, oil), bitter herbs (coriander, turmeric) help counter excess heat, itching and inflammation. Eczema (213) can also cause itching. It takes 3- 6 months to cure itching.

Jaundice

Jaundice is the yellowing of skin and or whites of the eyes caused by the accumulation of bilirubin in the blood. **Bilirubin** is the yellow pigment coloring of bile (digestion, fat emulsifier). **Bile**, produced by the liver is stored in the gall bladder, and released, into the small intestine via connecting ducts. Gallstones (page 223), hepatitis, alcoholism and or blood deficiency (includes anemia) tends to cause jaundice.

High protein, high fat foods (red meat, pork, turkey, chicken, fried foods, etc.) increase the production of bile. Too much bile tends to cause gallstones (can lodge in the gall bladder, ducts, cause obstruction, backup, reflux of bile, jaundice). Poor diet, including alcohol, sugar and overeating tends to cause liver and gall bladder disease.

The colder middle diet, meal plan, more fruits and vegetables, bitter herbs (gentian) and less animal protein, flesh, fried foods and alcohol is recommended, in addition to medical consultation and treatment.

22

"K- O" Diseases

Kidney Stones

Kidneys stones (renal calculi) are made from mineral salts and can occur anywhere in the urinary tract. Urine is generally saturated with uric acid, phosphates and calcium oxalate that normally remain suspended in solution (water) via a variety of chemical compounds designed to control urine pH (acid and alkaline balance). When the chemistry of these compounds becomes disturbed, altered, mineral substances, salts crystallize and clump together forming **stones**, which tend to

- Obstruct the flow of urine
- Cause pus and blood in the urine
- Cause frequent urination (odorous, cloudy), chills, fever and or profuse sweating,
- Cause great pain, radiating from the upper back down to the abdomen and groin

10% of Americans, mostly white men between ages 30-50, develop stones, at least once in their lifetime. **There are four kinds of stones**

- Calcium (composed of calcium oxalate)
- Uric acid (product of protein metabolism)
- Struvite (magnesium ammonium phosphate)
- Cystine

80% of all kidney stones are calcium oxalate. **Too much dairy** tends to cause high blood calcium levels, which increases the level of calcium in the urine.

Too much sugar (concentrated, natural or synthetic) increases blood sugar, which stimulates the pancreas to secrete insulin. Insulin lowers blood sugar while **increasing calcium elimination**, via urination.

Uric acid stones form when the volume of urine excreted is too low, and or uric acid levels, too high. High protein, diets produce excess uric acid (nitrogenous waste). High levels of uric acid also tend to produce gout.

Struvite stones tend to develop in women via recurring urinary tract infections.

The majority of kidney stones, **oxalic acid** are caused by too much protein, fat (including dairy), which is why they are more prevalent in white men, ages 30- 50 (tend to eat high protein, fat and starch diets). A malfunctioning parathyroid gland can also cause kidney stones.

The colder middle diet is recommended in addition to medical consultation. Fruits, vegetables (cooked, raw), radishes, spices (increase protein, fat digestion, thins the urine); magnesium (250- 500mg), **horsetail, corn silk, burdock** and **catnip tea**, and less animal, fried foods tend to reduce the formation of kidney stones. Too many spices can dry the urine and or irritate the bladder. Reduce alcohol, milk, yogurt, ice cream, etc.

Leukemia

There are two types of leukemia: acute and chronic. Acute leukemia is a malignant disease of the blood forming tissues (bone marrow, lymph nodes and spleen) characterized by uncontrollable production and accumulation of immature white blood cells (leukocytes). Leukocytes fight and destroy harmful bacteria and fungi.

Chronic leukemia is characterized by accumulation of mature leukocytes. The following are symptoms of acute and chronic leukemia.

- **Anemia**, fatigue, pallor, shortness of breath
- Excessive sweating, weight loss, fever
- Arthritic pain, enlarged lymph nodes
- Low immunity to colds, infections, **bleeding**

The symptoms of leukemia indicate chronic deficiency, coldness. The hotter middle diet, spices, bitter herbs and medical consultation is advised. Avoid sugar, tropical fruits, juices, soft dairy, alcohol and coffee.

Menopause

Menopause, cessation of menstruation usually occurs around ages forty-five to fifty-five. The following are symptoms commonly associated with menopause:

- Muscular and joint pain, osteoporosis
- Vaginal dryness, decreasing libido, fatigue
- Thin and dry skin, hair and nails, depression

Old age, excessive sex, caffeine and chronic blood deficiency via long-term low protein, low fat diets tend to accelerate the onset and severity of menopause. The middle diet and sage tea are recommended. More info (178- 9, 236- 237)

Menorrhagia and metrorrhagia

Uterine tumors and or cervical cancer via long-term high protein, high fat diets tend to cause metrorrhagia (uterine bleeding between periods) and menorrhagia (abnormally long or heavy menses. The colder middle diet is recommended, as is medical consultation.

Miscarriage

The fetus and uterus are a function of blood, nutrients, especially protein and fat (build, hold). Blood deficiency via long-term low protein, low fat diets and caffeine is a major cause. More info: pregnancy (263- 4)

Case history: A customer of mine, a woman in her early thirties had suffered four miscarriages. She was eating a macrobiotic diet (low protein, low fat). I diagnosed her condition as blood deficiency, anemia, not enough blood, protein and fat in the womb to hold her baby. I recommended the hotter middle diet, especially red meat, chicken and turkey 3- 4 times per week, Evening Primrose Oil (strengthens sexual organs) and Siberian ginseng (digestion) and told her to wait four months to rebuild her blood before trying to get pregnant. It takes four months, 120 days to rebuild blood. She now has two healthy boys.

Multiple Sclerosis

Multiple Sclerosis (MS) is a nervous system disorder caused by the **deterioration of the myelin sheath** (major, defining symptom). The myelin sheath is the fatty tissue that wraps and insulates nerve fibers. MS is often characterized as an autoimmune disease as the body's immune system malfunctions, producing antibodies that attack the myelin sheath, scarring the nerves distorting communication, producing the following symptoms:

- Dizziness, fatigue
- Blurred or double vision
- Tingling, numbness in the hands and feet
- Loss of balance and or muscular stiffness

In TCM, MS is generally characterized as a deficiency (deterioration) disease. Long-term low protein, low fat diet is the general cause. Protein and fat (especially animal) build thicken all structure, function. Too little, in the extreme, **thins, weakens all structure, function:** nerves, myelin sheath, balance, speech, vision, etc. especially in cold climates, which require, consume more substance, protein, fat, jing (to generate warmth, energy) accelerating the negative effects of blood deficiency.

MS (stage 6+ disease) is common in the US and Great Britain and less common, almost unheard of, in many Asian countries. Most Asians tend to eat the middle diet unlike many Americans who tend to eat **(1)** low protein, low fat (high dairy) and high carbohydrate (bread, salads, tropical fruits, juices, etc.) or **(2)** high protein, fat and starch and low vegetables, fruit.

MS tends to attack **women** between the ages of twenty-five and forty (menstruation) and is more common in the north than south.

Too much protein, fat, cholesterol and clogged arteries reduces circulation of blood, especially to the extremities: head, arms and legs causing fatigue, pain, inflammation, numbness, weakness, dizziness, slurred speech and or loss of balance, but **not** deterioration of the myelin sheath.

Deterioration of the myelin sheath is diagnosed medically with an MRI or spinal tap. Without this diagnosis, confirmation, the symptoms are more rheumatic, arthritic in nature, unlike the fixed and lasting symptoms of a deteriorated myelin sheath. Poor diet, chemical poisoning, pesticides, mercury, etc generally cause M.S. The hotter middle diet, meal plan is recommended for deficiency.

Nails

The epidermis (outer layer of skin) produces the nails, which are mostly **keratin** (protein) obtained via the diet. The nails protect the tips of the fingers and toes from external injury. It takes approximately **seven months** for the nails to grow from beginning to end. The following are common nail pathologies:

- Thin, dry, brittle, cracked
- Horizontal or vertical ridges
- Rounded, curved or spoon shaped
- White spots, hangnails, fungus

Poor diet weakens the nails.

- Long-term low protein, low fat diets, in the extreme, thin, weaken the blood (blood deficiency), which thins, weakens all structure, including the nails (thin, brittle, and cracked).

- Too many salads, tropical fruits, juices, sugar weaken digestion, decrease nutrient absorption, thin the blood.

- Too much protein, fat tends to overbuild, thicken, harden and yellow the nails.

The middle diet, meal plan adjusted accordingly is recommended.

- **Green vegetables** (cabbage, parsley celery, kale, broccoli, collard greens, etc.), high in minerals (calcium) raw and cooked help build the nails.

- Ground up **sesame seeds** (black, white, and organic if possible), 1-2 TBS per day sprinkled over food is effective in rebuilding nails, hair and skin.

- **For deficiency**, increase protein, fat (eggs, chicken, turkey, hard cheese, etc.).

- **Avoid, coffee, caffeine**, which tends to acidify the blood, and leach calcium and other minerals that build the nails, hair, bones, teeth, etc.

Fungal infections, worms and parasites (requires a medical diagnosis and or treatment) can also distort the nails. Sweet, damp conditions, foods nourish fungi.

- **Silica** supplements build hair, skin and nails

- Decrease raw vegetables, salads, tropical fruits, juices, cold drinks, dairy, ice cream, sugar, etc.

- Increase **seeds** (pumpkin, sesame, sunflower) and **spices** (cumin, coriander, fennel, turmeric, etc.).

- Try **vinegar** and water rinse and or **Australian Tea Tree oil** topically.

Nausea, vomiting

The throat, stomach, and small and large intestines are more or less **one long tube**. Digestive energy, food moves down the tube. If any part of the tube becomes blocked, a **back flow, reflux** of energy, food, fluids (burping, nausea, vomiting, etc.) tends to occur. It is no different from a clogged pipe that overflows.

Contaminated food, overeating (especially protein, fat and starch), indigestion, obesity, tight clothing, belts and bitter herbs (includes green tea) on an empty stomach constrict, narrow the stomach, small intestine slowing the downward movement of food causing it to collect, clog and rebel, move upwards.

Long-term low protein, low fat diets tend to weaken, slow digestion as does eating salads and fruits at the beginning of the meal. Bitter herbs (green tea) taken on an empty stomach may also be a factor, as they are cold, contracting (tightening) in nature.

The middle diet, meal plan adjusted accordingly is recommended. Eat less, smaller meals, if your problem is overeating. The stomach should be 3/4 full and 1/4 empty. Reduce dairy, processed grain, cold drinks, sodas, alcohol and overeating to improve digestion, movement of food. Loosen your belt when you eat, remain upright after eating and take a walk (to move food down). Do not lie down after a meal.

Spices (cardamom cumin, coriander, fennel, cayenne, ginger, etc.) increase digestion, movement of food, help relieve nausea and heartburn. Use in soups, vegetable dishes and desserts. Aloe vera in orange or apple juice may also help.

Numbness

Protein and fat build fuel and warm all structure function. Water, minerals, sugar, etc. cool, cleanse and moisten. Less blood, protein and fat numbs.

- Too little protein, fat, in the extreme, weakens, thins the blood (anemia, blood deficiency), which in turn, thins, weakens and dries all structure, function, especially the extremities hands, feet causing pain, numbness, coldness, inflammation, shaking, etc.

- Too much protein, fat can also cause numbness, via clogged arteries, which stagnate, reduce circulation, blood flow to the arms, legs.

- Environment can also be a factor. External cold (winter) decreases circulation to the hands and feet causing numbness.

The cold temperatures of winter, living in cold, damp basement, sleeping on the ground, etc. cause the body to drain, move blood from the arms, legs back to the chest, abdomen, where the vital organs are located. This leaves the limbs with less blood: numbness, coldness, shaking.

The middle diet, meal plan adjusted accordingly is recommended.   Do not overeat. More information: circulation (page 191)

Obesity

Obesity is an excess of body fat: **20% or greater** than normal body weight (adjusted for age, height, frame, sex, etc.). Poor diet, overeating (especially protein, fat and starch) and weak digestion are the primary causes.

Protein, fat and starch build thicken and clog the body. Too much not only increases body weight but also weakens digestion, which is the **ultimate fat burner**. Digestion burns breaks down and helps eliminate excess protein, fat, starch, sugar and water.

Weak digestion increases

- Waste as whatever food, nutrients, not digested, absorbed becomes waste that pastes and hardens the large intestine (bloating, dry stools, polyps)

- Blood clots, cholesterol and uric acid

- Arterial plaque, atherosclerosis

- Acne, warts, tumors

- Fatty growths, cellulite and edema in the thighs, hips, buttocks and abdomen

According to some doctors, obesity is a genetically predisposed hormonal condition that causes one to overeat. Certain foods trigger these hormones, excessive appetite but not negated when eliminating offending foods. This is total nonsense. Poor diet and lack of discipline are the true culprits.

If you took thousands of obese people and sent them to China to live for a year, where they could only eat rice, cooked vegetables, smaller amounts of protein and fat (fish, chicken, beans, etc.) and fruit with little or no dairy, what do you think would happen to their obesity and general health? Their obesity, excess fat would disappear while their overall health would improve. How many obese, native Chinese do you see versus obese Americans? You see very few. Less protein, fat, grain and less eating increases weight loss and longevity.

The middle diet, meal plan adjusted accordingly is recommended. Bitter herbs (page 54) help reduce fat. Reduce and or eliminate processed grains: bread, noodles, cookies, pretzels, chips, etc.), cooked potatoes (starchy, pasty) overeating and late night meals, snacks. Exercise, walking, especially after a meal helps move food down the small intestine (22 feet in length) increasing digestion and elimination. The more you digest, eliminate, the less you store.

The diet is easy, the mental part, more difficult. It requires will power to space, skip meals, reduce nighttime eating and stock fruit, vegetables, etc. instead of ice cream, beer, cookies, etc.

Just because you are hungry or have a sweet craving does not mean you have to eat the worst sweet. Trade up. **Snack** on apples, oranges, celery, carrots **Drink** juice or water when you feel hungry.

What is the worst thing that will happen to you if you do not eat sweets for one whole day? The answer is you will wake up the next day, feeling better and more confident. Remember all the negative aspects of your favorite negative, unhealthy foods, when you start to crave them

Osteoporosis

The bones are primarily **protein, fat and minerals** (calcium, magnesium, phosphorous, etc.). Osteoporosis (weakening, thinning of the bones) is a progressive disease that tends to attack women (80%) more than men. The thinning of bones is natural with age. Excessive bone loss is not.

Protein and fat are the glue, substance (not dairy, calcium) that holds bones, minerals together. **Long-term low protein, low fat diets, sugar and caffeine** weaken, thin the blood, which then thins the bones, as can the long-term use of blood thinners (page 129).

Many women tend to eat cold, damp, low protein, low fat (milk, yogurt cottage cheese, etc.) and high carbohydrate (fruits, juices, sugar, etc.) diets and caffeine, which thins the blood, bones, nerves, etc. Most men tend to eat high protein, high fat, which is a major reason why osteoporosis is more prevalent among women.

Thin blood (deficiency) despite a high dairy, calcium intake, thins, weakens the bones.

Menopause (dual decline in hormones and blood) may also be a cause, however, It is generally the underlying, long-term blood, protein and fat deficiency not estrogen deficiency that thins the bones. More info: menopause (pages 247)

Cold drinks, fruit juices and or salads eaten at the beginning of the meal, tend to dilute and weaken digestion, decreasing nutrient absorption, blood.

Acidic foods, sugar, caffeine, etc., in the extreme, tend to drain, **leech calcium and other minerals**, further weakening the bones.

Excessive sex also weakens, thins the bones as it drains jing (sexual essence, fundamental substance of the bones, marrow, brain, etc.).

Fish oil supplements help build the bones, brain, etc.

Leafy greens: cabbage, kale, broccoli, watercress and seaweeds (nori, kombu, etc.) contain more calcium than milk.

The middle diet, meal plan, adjusted accordingly is recommended. Reduce smoothies, cold drinks, sodas, etc. Avoid caffeine.

23

"P- R" Diseases

Pediatric Illnesses

Children (ages 1- 12) by nature are **cold, deficient** as their bodies are still developing. They tend to suffer cold, damp and deficient symptoms, diseases especially when fed a cold, damp diet.

- Abdominal bloating, gas, loose stools
- Mucous, phlegm, colds, sore throat, coughing
- Colic, pleurisy, pneumonia, whooping cough

Many children (American) tend to eat **cold, damp, diets** (milk, yogurt, ice cream, cereal, bread, pasta, tropical fruit, juices, sugar, cold, drinks, ice water, sodas, etc.). Cold damp diets

- Dilute, weaken and slow **digestion** (abdominal bloating, gas, burping) and **elimination** (loose stools, diarrhea, profuse urination) while reducing nutrient absorption, thinning the blood.

- Cool the body, lower body temperature, which in turn cools, dampens the lungs, throat, sinuses and ears with water, mucous, phlegm, etc.

The body is naturally warm and moist. Body temperature (98.6°) fueled by digestion, exercise, protein, fat, cooked foods, etc. heats, dries the body, especially the lungs, throat, mouth, sinuses, nose and ears, which lie above. Heat rises, moves up and out.

Lower body temperatures (less than 98.6°) via (1) blood deficiency, (2) cold, damp diet, climate, (3) under development and (4) chronic illness weaken, cool and **harden bodily fluids** in the lungs, bronchi, alveoli, throat, throat, sinuses and ears and into mucous, phlegm, cysts, etc. which

- Reduces gas, oxygen exchange
- Shortens the breath, asthma
- Coughing, hacking, snoring
- Earache, hearing loss
- Bacterial, viral infections

Bacteria, viruses and fungi thrive in stagnant, watery mediums. Trapped, stagnant water in ears, sinuses, lungs, etc. can attract, infect with bacteria, viruses, cause bronchitis, sinusitis, ear infections, colic, pleurisy and or pneumonia.

Building foods, protein, fat, cooked vegetables, **soups**, stews and **spices** stimulate digestion, increase energy, heat, circulation, body temperature, immunity, etc. A strong immune system incinerates, burns cold, damp pathogens (bacteria, viruses and fungi) via an increase in body temperature, fever and white blood cells. Fruits, juices, cold drinks and sugar, especially when eaten at the beginning of the meal cool, dilute and weaken digestion, reduce nutrient absorption, blood. Low protein, low fat and high carbohydrate diets, in the extreme weaken immunity. The worst foods, drinks for children, immunity are milk and cereal, ice cream, frozen yogurt, sugar, cold drinks, ice water, and sodas, especially if living in a cold climate.

Ear candles (wax and non-wax) help drain fluids from the ears, although wax candles may drip wax back into the ears. Check with your doctor first.

The cure is discipline. **Control** what your child eats at home. Do not stock junk, sweets. Keep a healthy kitchen (fruit, vegetables, bread, herb teas, juices, etc.). Practice (eat) what you preach if you want your children to follow your good not theoretical example. The good food, nutrition, health you serve at home, will eventually take over and outweigh cravings, tastes for junk food, drugs, peer pressure, etc. as they become more and more distasteful. Avoid vaccines preserved with mercury (may cause autism).

The middle diet, meal plan is recommended, two to three times per day, especially breakfast and lunch. Raspberry leaf tea helps treat diarrhea. Sample breakfasts (finish with herbal tea):

1. Vegetable omelet (3 vegetables), spices, toast, jelly
2. Chicken, rice; 3-5 cooked vegetables, spices, fruit
3. Cheese, cooked broccoli, raw carrots, celery, fruit
4. Turkey sandwich, 3-5 cooked vegetables, fruit
5. Beans, nuts, noodles, 3-5 vegetables, spices, fruit

Perspiration, sweating

The lungs control the skin, opening and closing of the pores. Perspiration is water that passes through the sweat glands in the skin. It helps cool the body via the elimination, sweating of excess heat, energy and waste, transported by water, sweat. **Too much** perspiration via excess heat, energy or **too little** via deficiency weakens, sickens the body.

Poor diet, extreme environment (excess heat, cold, humidity, etc.), obesity, tight clothing, chronic illness, etc. tend to increase or decrease perspiration, sweating.

Protein and fat build fuel all structure function, including opening and closing the pores.

- Too little weakens the body, lungs, and skin, causing the pores to be left open, leaking heat, energy and water: intermittent daytime or nighttime sweating. **Sage tea** helps counter night sweats. It also dries excess mucous in nose and lungs, stops bleeding, seminal discharges and mammary secretion.

- Too much protein, fat, fried foods, coffee and alcohol overheat the body: profuse perspiration

- Bacterial and viral infections can also cause excessive perspiration.

The middle diet, adjusted accordingly and or medical consultation is recommended

Plantar Fasciitis

Plantar Fasciitis (PF) is a common disease that usually occurs after age fifty. Its major symptom is excruciating pain in the heels, caused by **looseness and or inflammation of the plantar fascia,** and is usually worse upon rising, especially first thing in the morning. The pain never lets up. PF is sometimes, misdiagnosed as heel (calcaneus) spurs, which are not always painful. Poor diet, poor posture, misalignment and injury also cause PF.

The foot is not one bone but many. The plantar fascia (ligaments and other tissues) hold the heel (calcaneus) to the balls of the foot. The **heel** connects, forms a superior border, joint with the **talus** bone (connects, forms a joint with the **tibia**, lower leg bone), and a lower joint with the **navicular** bone (connects remaining bones in the feet).

All movable joints have the following symmetry, biology:

- **Ligaments** connect bone to bone.
- **Tendons** connect ligaments to **muscles**.
- **Nerves** electrical impulses connect, stimulate, contract (tighten) and expand (relax) the muscles, which pull, relax the tendons, ligaments and move the bones.
- **Blood, nutrients** build, fuel, moisten all structure, function.

Building nutrients: protein and fat thicken, build, fuel, hold and heat.

Too little protein, fat, in the extreme, tends to produce blood deficiency (anemia, thin blood), reduced circulation. Chronic blood deficiency, reduced circulation tends to dry, weaken, loosen, pain and inflame the joints, bones, ligaments, tendons, muscles, nerves, etc. in the arms, legs, hands and feet.

Too much protein and fat, especially animal, tends to clog and narrow the arteries (atherosclerosis), which also reduces circulation, blood, nutrient flow.

Blood deficiency and clogged arteries are the two major causes of most arthritic (inflammation of the joint) type diseases: PF, Rheumatoid Arthritis, Fibromyalgia, Restless Leg Syndrome, etc.

Case history: At age 54, I developed excruciating pain in my heels (started in right heel before progressing into the left). The pain was worse, especially upon rising, first thing in the morning or after sitting or lying down for any extended period, but did seem to get better with movement, exercise (improved circulation).

In the beginning, when I first started suffering, I thought I was doomed, just getting older (50's), and suffering what naturally came with age. I did see a doctor who told me there was an operation to correct it: cut open heals and sew the loose ligaments together. **Loose ligaments** told me my condition was a circulatory disorder, as my blood was **not circulating fully** to my legs, feet, ligaments, etc., which, in turn caused looseness, pain. Blood, protein and fat holds all tissues together. Lack of blood, nutrients causes pain, weakness, looseness, etc. The cause was clogged arteries due to past high protein, high fat diet.

My diet, which I had changed thirty years ago, did not totally cleanse, unclog my arteries. I needed to do better, thin my diet. I eliminated all animal protein except turkey while increasing Swiss cheese, beans, nuts and seeds. The rest of the diet was white basmati rice, noodles, vegetables, cooked and raw (cabbage, celery), spices (fennel), fruit (apples), peppermint tea and bitter herbs (golden seal) while avoiding the nightshade family: cooked potatoes, tomatoes (aggravate arthritis). I also ate less, spaced and or skipped meals. Dinner was always small. Fruit became my nighttime snack.

It took 7-8 months of continual pain, suffering and limping to figure it out and an additional three months to cure, as in 100% no pain, no recurrence, just long satisfying walks (2- 5 miles per day). My blood pressure and weight also significantly decreased. Poor diet caused my Plantar Fasciitis.

Poor posture, misalignment of bones, high arches, inappropriate shoes, injury or chronic illness can also be a cause.

Pneumonia

Pneumonia is inflammation of the lungs caused by bacterial infection. Extreme cold, damp diets or climate can attack, cool and dampen the lungs with excess fluids (water, mucous, phlegm). Excess fluids not only obstruct and shorten the breath but also foster bacterial growth:

- Coughing, hacking, painful breathing, headaches
- Expectoration of thick sputum
- Inflammation, fever, chest pain

Pneumonia, pleurisy, asthma and bronchitis tends to attack children and the elderly, especially when they eat cold, damp diets and or live in a cold, damp climate. The hotter middle diet for cold, damp is recommended as is medical consultation and or treatment. More info: Lungs (131- 8)

Pregnancy

Blood, **protein and fat** build and fuel the ovaries, uterus, hormones, ovum, sperm, fetus, etc. Pregnancy requires additional protein, fat as you are eating, building, for two. Anything less, shortens or miscarries.

Too little, in the extreme, reduces, thins the blood

- **Thin blood** thins the hair, skin, bones, sexual organs: amenorrhea (little or no period), infertility, miscarriage, short-term pregnancy

Too much can also prevent fertility, pregnancy, via

- Tumors, excessive tissue in, or around the ovaries, fallopian tubes and or uterus

Many women tend to eat cold, damp, low protein, low fat (milk, yogurt, cottage cheese, ice cream, etc.) and high carbohydrate (salads, fruits, juices, shakes, smoothies, sodas, sugar) diets, drink coffee (bad for pregnancy).

Cold, damp diets to weaken digestion reduce nutrient absorption, blood, energy, body temperature. **Lower body temperatures cool, dampen and clog** the body, **ovaries and fallopian tubes** with excess fluids, slowing and or preventing the dissension of the egg, leading to ectopic pregnancy (this is one cause).

Low protein, low fat diets generally benefit those suffering from high protein, high fat diseases, not those trying to get and stay pregnant.

The **hotter middle diet**, for blood deficiency is recommended, in addition to:

- **Siberian ginseng** strengthens spleen, digestion

- **Evening primrose, black currant oil** and **American red raspberry lea**f tea nourish, strengthen the reproductive organs.

- **Fenugreek** seeds (gruel) improve milk flow.

- **Laxative and bitter herbs should be avoided** cleansing, downward moving

- Check with your doctor first.

Male fertility: Low protein, low fat diets, caffeine and smoking decrease testosterone, sperm, erections, fertility and sexual desire. High protein, high fat diets, especially animal flesh, increase sexual desire and heart attacks,

Pre Menstrual Syndrome

Pre Menstrual Syndrome (PMS) is a series of symptoms, physical and mental that tends to occur several days prior to the onset of menstruation. Poor diet is the general cause; as it tends to slow, weaken, decrease digestion, elimination, nutrient absorption, blood and circulation:

- Abdominal bloating, swelling of the breasts
- Fatigue, water retention, headache, acne
- Backache, joint pain, cramps, depression,
- Anxiety, mood swings, outbursts of anger

The majority of these symptoms indicate chronic blood and chi deficiency and stagnation

Many women tend to eat low protein, low fat and high carbohydrate diets. Protein and fat build, fuel. Low protein, low fat (soft dairy, beans, etc.) diets, in the extreme, **thin the blood**, which in turn, thins, weakens and slows all structure, function, producing fatigue, joint pain, backache, acne, depression, anxiety, mood swings, cramps, headaches, etc

Too many tropical fruits, juices, shakes, cold drinks (soda, ice water, etc.), tend to dilute, weaken digestion slowing and stagnating the movement of food and fluids (abdominal bloating, gas, loose stools, water retention).

Too much protein, fat can also be a cause. The liver stores, cleanses (removes excess protein, fat, cholesterol) and releases the blood. High protein, fat diets, in the extreme, thicken the blood, which clogs, weakens the liver. Less protein, fat is removed, more stays, and thickens the blood (clots, high cholesterol).

Thick high protein, high fat liver blood passes directly into the uterus, and in the extreme, tends to cause

- PMS, menstrual clots
- Dysmenorrhea, endometriosis

The middle diet, meal plan, adjusted accordingly is recommended. Reduce grain, especially processed.

Prostate, inflammation and cancer

The prostate, located below the urinary bladder, is the doughnut shaped male, sex gland that encircles the urethra. It stores and releases semen mixed with prostatic fluids into the urethra. There are **three major pathologies**

- Inflammation
- Enlargement (benign prostatic hypertrophy BPH)
- Cancer

Poor diet, bacterial infection and excessive sex tend to weaken, sicken the prostate.

Prostate symptoms

- Impotence, premature ejaculation
- Difficulty urinating, interrupted stream
- Unbearable urge to urinate
- Pus, blood in the urine

High protein, high fat diets, especially animal, fried foods and overeating, in the extreme, thicken and clog the blood, arteries, prostate, etc. causing

- Pain, inflammation, tumors and or cancer

The colder middle diet is recommended in addition to

- **Bitter herbs**

- **Pumpkin seeds** (high in zinc and essential fatty acids) help reduce the size of the prostate. Prostate cancer is virtually unknown in certain areas of China where they eat pumpkin seeds one handful per day, and a low protein, low fat diet.

- **Saw palmetto**

- **Parsley tea**

Medical consultation and or treatment may be necessary.

Psoriasis

Psoriasis is a painful chronic skin disorder characterized by **dry, red, scaly skin** covering the scalp, genitalia, skin, back, etc. that tends to alternate between exacerbation (hot) and remission. It is a "hot" disease, caused in general by too much building, protein, fat, especially animal flesh and fried foods, in addition to starch, alcohol and sweets.

Too much protein, fat, in the extreme, saturates the blood, arteries with excess protein, fat, which eventually overflows into the skin, hardening, drying, reddening, etc.

Case history I counseled a young man (38) with severe psoriasis: dry, scaly, flaky and inflamed skin on his head, face, back, etc. He was also overweight and constantly scratching. His original diet was high protein, fat (red meat, pork, fried foods, etc.). I advised the colder middle diet, especially raw vegetables and fruit.

In seven months, his face, head and back completely cleared up. He also lost 60# and looked 15 years younger.

Rashes

Excess heat and dampness (kapha) via diet, climate, disease (measles, chicken pox and rubella), diaper rash and or genetics tend to cause rashes: raised, reddening of the skin in red spots or generalized areas

Too much protein, fat (oil) and flour tends to paste, thicken, dampen and clog the small and large intestines. Overtime the body (98.6°F) cooks heats this paste (damp), weight causing the intestines and the body to overheat, and in the extreme, pass, rise, move up and out into skin, back, shoulders, neck chest, face, groin and or armpits resulting in general reddening that maybe dry, flaky and or moist. Moist groin rashes are an extreme form of damp (kapha) heat (pitta) that collects in the center of the body. Dampness by nature is cold, but can heated by body temperature (98.6°F) turned into damp heat.

Too much protein, fat and sugar tends to clog and overheat the liver and gall bladder, which tends to cause **neck, armpit and groin rashes** (damp, red and oily). All excess sugar (includes fruit) is turned into fat.

Dietary rashes are a chronic, stage 5 disease taking months to develop and consequently months of good eating to cure. Left untreated these types of rashes may turn into psoriasis (stage 6). The colder middle diet, meal plan (less grains, nuts and oily foods) is recommended. Vary the diet and herbs according to results. Topical treatments include turmeric cream and aloe vera gel.

Dietary rashes, reduce
- Salty, sour and pungent tastes, coffee, smoking
- Animal, fried foods, oil, alcohol, hot spices
- Meat, dairy, nuts, processed grains

Dietary rashes, increase
- Sweet and bitter tastes
- Whole grains, beans, raw vegetables, fruit

Spices (mild, especially coriander), bitter herbs, low protein, low fat and raw and cooked foods help dry, drain and eliminate dampness, rashes.

Restless Leg Syndrome

Restless Leg Syndrome (RLS) is a condition in which the legs develop painful cramps, twitch, jerk, and or kick involuntarily while lying in bed, day or night (wakefulness, insomnia). Poor diet is one cause.

Long-term blood, protein, fat deficiency and or clogged arteries tend to cause poor circulation. Poor circulation reduces, decreases blood, nutrient flow, especially to the legs, bones, ligaments, tendons, muscles, nerves, causing

- Dryness, pain, inflammation
- Weakness, cramps, numbness
- Rheumatoid Arthritis, Restless Leg Syndrome
- Peripheral Artery Disease (PAD)

Protein and fat build, fuel, stimulate all structure, function. Too little weakens and thins the blood. Thin blood (blood deficiency), in the extreme, reduces circulation, thins, dries, pains, inflames, numbs and weakens the bones, ligaments, tendons, muscles and nerves, especially in the extremities: head, arms, legs.

Long-term high animal protein, fat diets thicken the blood (clots, high cholesterol) and clog, narrow the arteries (plaque, atherosclerosis), reducing circulation, to the arms, legs, bones, muscles: dryness, pain, inflammation, twitching jerking, numbness, RLS, etc

Reduced, interrupted blood flow, nutrients to the legs, causes the muscles, tendons to occasionally twitch, jerk or become numb, especially when lying down, as the body, heart, lungs, etc. is less active, pumping, circulating less blood to the extremities.

For cold, deficiency (anemia, fatigue, pallor, etc.) the hotter middle diet (more animal protein, turkey, chicken, eggs, hard cheese, etc. less raw foods, sugar) is recommended. For hot, excessive (high cholesterol, clogged arteries, etc.), the colder middle diet (vegetarian) is recommended.

Restless Leg Syndrome cold, deficient
Stage 1 Diet: long-term low protein, low fat, high carb
Stage 2 Digestion: abdominal bloating, gas
Stage 3 Elimination: loose stools, constipation
Stage 4 Blood deficiency: anemia, pallor, fatigue
Stage 5 Poor circulation: RLS, RA, PAD

Restless Leg Syndrome hot, overbuilt
Stage 1 Diet: long-term high protein, fat, starch
Stage 2 Digestion: abdominal bloating, gas
Stage 3 Elimination: constipation
Stage 4 Blood stagnation: clogged arteries
Stage 5 Poor circulation: Restless Leg, RA, PAD

24

"S" Diseases

Sex, reproduction

Sex is a two-edged sword. On one hand, it is procreative and highly pleasurable. On the other, it is the kiss of death, aging process, more so for men than women.

Sex, masturbation, orgasm releases jing (sexual essence, sperm, ovum). **Jing** is the body's primary substance, fuel that transforms into the sexual organs, marrow, bones, brain, spinal chord and original chi (fuels all function). It is the fountain of youth when full and the specter of old age, death, in its decline. Decline starts soon after sexual maturity and varies according to the individual. Proper diet, exercise and sexual control can slow its decline.

Jing depletion
- Weak bones, teeth, knees, lower back pain
- Infertility, incontinence, forgetfulness, fear
- Dry skin, hair loss
- Weak vision, hearing loss, insomnia

Causes
- Old age, chronic illness, workaholic
- Excessive sex, smoking, long-term insomnia
- Caffeine, alcohol, drugs, amphetamines
- Long-term anemic diet
- Extreme hot climate

The body is naturally hot. Normal body temperature (98.6°F) heats, dries and thins bodily fluids. Colder body temperatures (<98.6°F) via long-term cold, damp diets (milk, cottage cheese, ice cream, fruits, juices, cold drinks) or climate, weaken, cool, lower body temperature. Lower body temperatures cool harden fluids in the lungs, nose, throat, sinuses, uterus and vagina into

- Mucous, phlegm, cysts, fibroids, cellulite
- Yeast and bladder infections

Chronic, long-term **blood, protein and fat deficiency** thins, weakens, dries all structure, function: **reproduction**

- Impotence, premature ejaculation
- Amenorrhea, infertility, miscarriage
- short-term pregnancy, insufficient lubrication
- Inability to orgasm, lack of sexual desire

Too much animal protein, fat, in the extreme, thickens the blood (clots, high cholesterol) in the **uterus, vagina**

- Dysmenorrhea, endometriosis
- Pelvic inflammatory disease, tumors, cancer

Thick blood clogs the arteries (plaque) reducing circulation, blood to the **ovaries, uterus and penis**

- Infertility miscarriage, short-term pregnancy
- Impotence, premature ejaculation

Too much protein, fat, especially animal flesh also tends to increase **masculinity, body hair, aggression and sexual desire in both sexes**, which is why many religions recommend vegetarianism, to reduce, cool sexual fire, desire.

Sexual desire is the forbidden fruit as its short-lived pleasure comes at a high cost: premature aging. Relationships, love based on sex rarely last.

The **sexual strength** of man comes not from size but from jing (sexual essence) and blood (nutrients). Jing is limited. You get one fuel tank at birth. The faster you use it up the faster you age, weaken. Sex (orgasm, ejaculation) consumes, burns the most jing, which is why men are advised to restrain, avoid the orgasm, **start but do not finish** to conserve jing. The more jing a man saves the longer and stronger his erections and time of lovemaking. The only time man should ejaculate is in the pursuit of children. Orgasm is less damaging to women, due in large part to menstruation.

The middle diet, meal plan, royal jelly, adjusted accordingly, in addition to sexual control and or celibacy is recommended. Eat lesser animal, more plant. Reduce *avoid coffee, caffeine,* smoking and alcohol, which are extremely weakening, drying. Reduce sex to discover the more important things (spirituality) in life.

Shaking, Tremors

Blood, protein and fat builds, fuels, strengthens and holds the muscles, tendons, bones, nerves, etc. Reduced circulation, blood, nutrients via clogged arteries or blood deficiency, in the extreme, weakens, loosens, dries, shakes, trembles and pains the muscles, tendons, ligaments, and nerves (Parkinson's disease).

High protein, high fat diets, in the extreme, thicken the blood, clogs the arteries and reduces circulation. Low protein, low fat diets, in the extreme, reduce, thin and weaken the blood (blood deficiency)

Chronic blood deficiency and reduced circulation thin, dries and weakens all structure, function. **Shaking, trembling and paralysis** indicate **deficiency**, lack of holding (yang) as well as **air, wind** (vata) in the vessels (arteries, meridians). Long-term shaking, tremors indicates chronic disease. Consult with a doctor.

The middle diet, meal plan adjusted accordingly and skullcap is recommended.

Extreme cold weather is also a cause, as blood naturally retreats, moves back from the limbs to the chest, abdomen to protect and nourish vital organs leaving the limbs with less blood, energy, holding power, etc. causing air, wind: shaking, trembling, etc.

Sinusitis

The sinuses: **frontal** (above the eyes), **ethmoid** (either side of the nose and above the nose), **sphenoid** (behind the bridge of the nose) and **maxillary** (inside the cheekbones) are air-filled naturally moist (mucous) pockets connected to the nose and throat by passageways designed to conduct air and drain excess mucous. Moisture helps keep the sinuses cleans, free of debris.

Too much moisture (water, mucous, phlegm) tends to block, dry, pressurize and inflame the nasal sinuses: sinusitis. Too little also inflames.

Sinusitis has two classifications: **acute and chronic**. Bacterial and viral infections tend to cause acute (rapid onset) sinusitis. Small growths, injury to the nasal bones, smoking, pollution and or allergies (hay fever) tend to cause chronic sinusitis.

Too much moisture in the sinuses not only obstructs, narrows, but also providing the breeding ground for **bacteria and viruses,** which thrive (inflame, infect) in stagnant, fluid mediums. Cold, damp diets or climates, in the extreme, tend to cool the body, thicken bodily fluids in the lungs, sinuses, etc.

Body temperature (98.6°F) and digestion (three meals per day) normally heats, dries the body, especially the lungs, head, which lie above. Heat rises.

Long-term cold, damp low protein, low fat diets (milk, soft cheese, ice cream, tropical fruits, juices, smoothies and cold drinks) weaken digestion, decrease nutrient absorption, blood, energy, body temperature, as does overexposure to extreme cold weather.

Colder body temperatures (<98.6°F) cool and thicken fluids in the lungs, bronchi, alveoli, throat, sinuses, nose, breast, into excess mucous (thick water), phlegm (thick mucous), cysts, etc., in the same way colder temperatures (night, winter, etc.) thicken and harden water in the air into the morning dew, rain, snow and ice.

The hotter middle diet for cold, damp is recommended. Protein, fat, cooked foods and hot spices stimulates digestion, heats the body. Spices dry mucous, phlegm, edema, etc., and are antibacterial. Reduce dairy, processed grains, cold drinks.

Case history: One of my employees was suffering from sinusitis (inflammation of the sinuses). Her long-term vegetarian diet (milk, yogurt, ice cream, grains, salads, tropical fruits, juices, cold drinks, etc.) was cold, damp. I recommended the hotter middle diet, spices. Spices heat the body, increase blood flow. Blood moistens dryness, inflammation. Her condition cured.

Skin diseases

The skin builds up (anabolism) and breaks down (catabolism) largely according to food, nutrients: building and cleansing. Building nutrients (protein, fat) build, thicken, fuel and heat. Cleansing nutrients, foods (water, minerals, fruits, vegetables) reduce, cleanse, cool and moisten. Too much or too little building, in the extreme tends to cause skin disease via (a) too much (thick, hard) or (b) too little (thin, loose) skin. There are only two dietary skin diseases.

- Hot, excess (high protein, fat): acne, psoriasis
- Cold, deficient (low protein, fat): eczema

Acne (page 159) is an **inflammatory (hot)** disease of the sebaceous glands primarily affecting the face, shoulders and back producing raised, red lesions, pustules, blackheads, etc. Sebaceous glands located throughout the body in the dermis (layer of skin below the epidermis, outer layer) secrete sebum (oily liquid) that helps the body retain heat, while also moistening the skin, hair. **Psoriasis** (267) is also a hot, high protein, high fat disease.

Too much protein, fat, especially animal, fried foods (oil, pizza, lasagna, cookies, chips, fries, etc.) saturates and thickens the blood (clots, high cholesterol) and in the extreme, overflows into the skin, face, neck and back causing

- **Acne** raised red lesions, pustules, blackheads, hard painful, oily pimples, boils. pus

- **Psoriasis** itchy dry, red, scaly, flaky skin covering the scalp (dandruff, flakes), genitalia, skin and back

- **Warts, moles, tumors**

- **Shingles**

Too little protein, fat weakens, thins the blood (blood deficiency). **Too many** juices, cold drinks dilute, weaken digestion, reducing nutrient absorption, blood. Chronic blood deficiency tends to weaken, break apart the skin, muscles, etc. Eczema (page 213) is generally a cold, damp (kapha) and deficient symptom, disease.

- **Eczema** dry, cracked, red (red spots, splotches, bleeding), blister like formations that **weep**, release fluid before forming a crust, scale or flake.

- Exposed capillaries, blue veins, sagging skin

For "hot" acne, psoriasis, the colder middle diet is recommended, and for "cold" eczema, the hotter middle diet. **Calendula oil** is great for burns, scarring and wounds. I once suffered a large second-degree burn on my chest. I washed it with salt water, and then put calendula on it for several days. It never scarred.

Skin diseases cold, deficient
Stage 1 Diet: long-term low protein, low fat, high carb
Stage 2 Digestion: abdominal bloating, gas
Stage 3 Elimination: loose stools
Stage 4 Blood deficiency: partial facial flushing, red spots
Stage 5 Poor circulation: eczema, exposed capillaries

Skin diseases hot, overbuilt
Stage 1 Diet: long-term high protein, fat, starch
Stage 2 Digestion: abdominal bloating, gas
Stage 3 Elimination: constipation
Stage 4 Blood stagnation: raised, red, oily pimples
Stage 5 Poor circulation: warts, acne, psoriasis, itching

Sleep apnea

Sleep apnea is a severe form of **insomnia** (239) characterized by **snoring** and extreme **irregular breathing** throughout the night that sometimes stops the breath for 1-2 minutes, causing oxygen deprivation, sudden wakefulness, gasping for air. It is a chronic lung (includes nose, throat and sinuses) condition generally caused by excess mucous, high blood pressure and or obesity. Diet, herbs and medicated, aromatic (spicy) nose strips help drain, open the sinuses.

The lungs are naturally moist. Water, moisture facilitates the exchange of water-soluble gases (oxygen and carbon dioxide).

Too much moisture (mucous, phlegm) weakens, decreases the exchange, causing

- Oxygen deprivation, shortness of the breath
- Coughing, hacking (clearing of the throat)
- Snoring, sinusitis, insomnia

Too little fluid and smoking tends to cause dryness

- Dry lungs, throat, shortness of breath, coughing.

Body temperature (98.6°F) and digestion heat the body and regulate (thin) bodily fluids (water, mucous, etc.). Long-term cold, damp, low protein, low fat (milk, yogurt, ice cream, etc.) and high carbohydrate (tropical fruits, juices, smoothies, shakes, cold drinks (soda, ice water, etc.) diets, overexposure to cold, damp climates (winter, air conditioning, sleeping in a cold, damp basement, etc.) and chronic illness weaken, cool, **lower body temperature,** which cools, dampens the body.

Cold condenses. In nature, colder temperatures harden moisture, water in the air or on the ground into the morning dew, rain, snow (white flakes) and or ice. In the body, colder temperatures thicken and harden fluids in the lungs, throat, sinuses into mucous, phlegm causing

- shortness of breath, coughing
- Snoring, sleep apnea

The **hotter middle diet** for cold, damp sleep apnea is recommended. Spices contain essential oils that are hot, drying (decrease dampness, mucous), antiviral, antibacterial and aromatic, opening up the sinuses, breathing passages, increasing air, oxygen exchange.

The **colder middle diet** for the hot, overbuilt, obese sleep apnea is recommended. Obesity, clogged intestines also closes the nostrils, restricts breathing, etc., which is why it is good to get up and move around, have a glass of juice, go to the bathroom if you cannot sleep.

Snoring

Excess fluids (mucous, phlegm) and dryness in the lungs, throat, sinuses, nose, obstructs the nasal passages, breath causing snoring, hacking, etc. in an attempt to dislodge, expectorate the obstruction.

Too little protein, fat; too many cold, damp foods, drinks (ice cream, milk, salads, juices, cold drinks) or overexposure to cold weather tends to lower body temperature, which cools and hardens fluids in the nose, sinuses, etc into excess mucous, phlegm.

Smoking dries, narrows and obstructs the lungs, throat, nose, sinuses and cause snoring, as can obesity (excess weight overheats, dries and tightens the body.

The middle diet adjusted accordingly is recommended. Excess mucous and phlegm takes weeks, months to form, and dissolve.

Sore throat

Blood and body fluids nourish, moisten the throat. Decreased blood flow via (1) blood, protein and fat deficiency, (2) clogged arteries, (3) overexposure to cold (winter, a/c) and (4) hot weather (heat, dryness) and or (5) smoking dries, irritates the throat. The middle diet, adjusted according is recommended plus

- **Peppermint** tea is soothing to a sore throat and helps counter the drying effects of smoking.
- Bayberry, burdock, coriander, licorice

Sweaty Hands and feet

I once counseled a woman who was sweating profusely in her feet and hands. It was summer. The A/C was off and it was 80°F outside and inside. There was an operation to correct it. Her son (18), who had the same condition, had the operation (removed sweat glands in hands, feet), which while curing the condition in the hands, feet, caused heavy sweating in other areas of the body. I asked her what she ate for breakfast and lunch. She had a grilled cheese sandwich and coffee for breakfast, and meat and rice for lunch. Her diet was hot, thick and dry: too much protein, fat, starch and coffee, and not enough fruit, vegetables. Her condition was worse in summer. Her body was too thick, overheated, causing profuse perspiration, sweating (to eliminate excess heat, energy) via the extremities.

I recommended the colder middle diet and sage tea.

25

"T- Z" Diseases

Teeth

The teeth, bone, nerves are built fueled and cleansed by blood, nutrients. The correct balance, diet keeps the body, teeth, nerves, etc. healthy. The incorrect balance, foods (sugar, alcohol, drugs, etc.) and overeating weaken decay, inflame and infect the teeth, nerves.

Pain in the teeth, gums occurs when a cavity, decay and infection penetrate into the nerve. It is the infected nerve and not the decayed tooth (enamel, dentin-covered-pulp) that causes pain. Dental caries (cavities), pain, abscesses are treated with drilling, fillings, root canals, extractions, antibiotics, etc.

Too much sugar (concentrated, processed, natural, white, brown, fructose, maple syrup, etc.), protein, fat, oil and sweets (cookies, pastries, ice cream, chocolate, soda, etc.) nourishes bacteria that infect, inflame, pain the nerves and or cause abscesses (accumulation of pus caused by the breakdown of tissues).

Proper diet, natural foods (fruit, vegetables, nuts, seeds, cheese, spices, herbs, etc.), increased flossing, brushing (xylitol toothpaste) and or Water Pick with warm water, sage and peppermint oil can help prevent and or cure, depending on severity and ability to discipline one's own diet, most tooth, nerve infections. The cure, stopping of the infection is temporary, only lasts as long as the corrections last, as poor diet will restart the infection.

Too much sugar, oil, fat, processed grains etc. also weaken and inflame the stomach and large intestine, whose meridians (energetic pathways) pass through the mouth, gums. The large intestine and stomach are energetically active from 3 A.M. to 7 A.M. Pain in the teeth during this time indicates stomach and large intestine dysfunction, which may inflame, bleed the gums. Tooth pain that lessens, goes away later in the morning and early afternoon generally indicates that the nerves are not fully damaged and may be restored, as long as you eat well.

Simple foods: fruit, vegetables, spices, herbs fight, prevent and heal infection. Eat yogurt instead of ice cream. Eat raw vegetables (celery, carrots, lettuce, etc.) and fruit (apples, oranges, pineapple, etc.) instead of bread, cookies, crackers, chips, candy. Everything, including the nerves, infection and disease builds up and breaks down. Infection, tooth decay, etc. will diminish; go away if you stop feeding it, eat well.

It is still wise to regularly see a dentist and get regular cleanings and or treatment. Most dentists probably do not believe that infected nerves can be healed, restored through diet.

Case history: In 2003, I was living in Issaquah, WA. In the summer, I used to hike in the mountains, and go swimming in the river at Twin Falls. Mountain water is incredibly cold, even in the summer. No one can stay in more than twenty minutes. While swimming, I got water in my ears and the next day I developed a severe tooth and gum ache that inflamed my right upper gums and teeth. I tried to cure it naturally. Nothing worked. A week later, **I went to a dentist**. He and his partner were confused as to which tooth, root was decayed, infected, as the x-rays were inconclusive

They tested each tooth many times, but with all the medication, I could not tell which one was infected. They finally settled on one tooth and did a root canal ($1300) and new crown. They both thought the tooth would ooze blood, pus once they opened it up. Nothing came out, except a few drops.

The next day the pain came back in full. They had drilled, killed the wrong tooth, nerve. Fortunately, I was motivated, able to nullify the pain via acupuncture, peppermint oil (several drops, 5- 10 times per day, swish around the infected tooth, gum), turmeric, sage tea and Ibuprofen (anti-inflammatory) four tablets every 4- 5 hours). I did not go back to the dentist.

For the next few years, the pain, inflammation, looseness, etc. in my gums, teeth would come and go, with my diet. Three years later, it turned into an abscess, a big white pimple on the side of my gums. I would pop the abscess (it would squirt out with force) and the pain would lessen. Developing an abscess motivated me to eat better.

I eliminated pretzels, chips, cookies, candies, sweets, chocolate and alcohol. I continued using tea tree oil (anti-fungal), peppermint oil (antibacterial), xylitol (antibacterial) toothpaste, myrrh, raspberry leaf tea and Ibuprofen (when needed), in addition to daily flossing, which eliminated, cured the infection, abscess (as long as I ate well). Once I started eating poorly, the infection, pain, loose teeth would automatically come back.

Years later, another tooth, root, nerve on the opposite side became infected. I had x-rays, dental examination but refused the suggested root canals. I was able once again to cure via diet, peppermint oil, Ibuprofen, Water Pick, flossing, etc.

Getting better usually occurs in stages that may take days or weeks to occur. The healing process, slow but methodical, varies with the individual, according to his her discipline. If you cure it (pain goes away) once you can cure it again. If you cannot, see a dentist.

Tinnitus

Tinnitus is ringing (humming sound) in the ears. It can have several causes:

- Hearing loss, wax buildup, spicy foods, caffeine
- Obesity, hypertension (high blood pressure)

The dietary causes are correctable via elimination, reduction of caffeine, spices, overeating, etc.

Hearing loss and wax buildup generally requires a doctor.

Ear candles or few drops of garlic oil or hydrogen peroxide in the ears helps eliminate wax buildup. Check with your doctor

In TCM, there are two types of tinnitus

- **Loud ringing** (hot) is associated with liver congestion, atherosclerosis and high blood pressure via too much protein, fat, and starch.

- **Low ringing** (cold) is associated with kidney yin deficiency via excessive sex, blood deficiency and caffeine.

The middle diet, meal plan, adjusted accordingly, is recommended. There are also normal, healthy astral, musical "ringing" sounds.

Tumors

Uncontrollable growth, cell proliferation of tissue tends to cause tumors, **benign** (harmless) and **malignant** (deadly, cancerous). Most tumors are caused by high protein, high fat diets, especially animal (red meat, pork, etc.) and fried foods, which thicken the blood (clots, high cholesterol) too much causing tumors and or cancer. Fruits, vegetables, spices, less protein, fat and eating decrease blood, cholesterol, tumors, etc. Everything, including disease requires food. The best way to prevent and or cure disease is to stop feeding it.

The colder middle diet, meal plan is recommended. Reduce or eliminate animal flesh (red meat, chicken, turkey). Increase fruit and vegetables, raw (beets) and cooked Seventy percent of the diet should be vegetables, fruit. Tumors are easy to break down. Check with your doctor first to determine the severity of your tumor, cancer. There is nothing wrong with drugs, surgery and radiation, especially if it saves your life. Going the natural way requires a lot of faith, discipline and ability to stand some pain.

Urinary Tract Infection (cystitis)

The kidneys filter and convert nitrogenous wastes from the bloodstream into urea, urine temporarily stored in the urinary bladder and later eliminated via ureters and urethra (hollow tubes). Diet and biology determine viscosity (texture, thickness), chemistry (electrolyte, acid and alkaline balance) and efficiency of urination.

Urinary bladder infections: cystitis (bladder infection), urethritis (infection of urethra) and acute pyelonephritis (kidney infection) are more common in women.

Eighty-five percent of all urinary bladder infections are caused by **bacterium** via

- Diet
- Sexual intercourse
- Elimination (because of close proximity of urethra to anus, increases potential fecal bacteria transmission)

Thick urine via (1) high protein, fat, cholesterol diets or (2) too many cold, damp foods, drinks (milk, yogurt, soft cheese, ice cream, salads, juices, sodas, cold drinks and sugar) tends to move slowly, and can clog the tubes, making urination difficult, painful, burning, frequent and or urgent. It also invites, tends to foster **bacterial** growth, contamination, urinary tract infection, which is why spices and cranberry juice are used, both of which counter, kill bacterial growth.

Pregnant women often develop bladder infections, as the baby, fetus, and abdomen, eventually grow and presses upon the bladder restricting or stagnating the flow of urine.

The middle diet, meal plan, adjusted accordingly, is recommended.

- **Cranberry** juice or concentrate (in pill, capsule form) are a popular cure for most bladder infections. Cranberries are acidic help burn; dissolve noxious bacteria, dampness while also thinning the urine, making it easier to pass.

- **Spices** cumin, coriander and fennel, in vegetable soup increase digestion, reduce cold, damp and help thin the urine. Most spices are antibacterial.

- **Bitter herbs** should be avoided.

Consult with a doctor, as bladder infections may require antibiotics.

Varicose Veins

Veins transport blood. Valves within the veins prevent back flow. Poor diet, alcohol, excessive sitting; lack of exercise, obesity, pregnancy, heavy lifting and or poor circulation via malfunctioning valves via blood deficiency or clogged arteries tends to cause varicose veins

- Abnormally enlarged, bulging, lumpy
- Bluish in color

Low protein, fat diets, in the extreme, tend to thin, reduce the blood, circulation, especially to the lower extremities, legs causing the blood to stagnate, pool and outline the veins, giving the skin a bluish tint. Obesity and sedentary lifestyle also tend to cause varicose veins. The middle diet, meal plan adjusted accordingly is recommended, in addition to exercise. Reduce alcohol, coffee, caffeine, which are weakening, drying.

TCM, acupuncture lances, bleeds varicose veins. Consult with a physician or acupuncturist. Washing, soaking with apple cider vinegar may also help shrink veins.

Weight Loss

The body builds up and breaks down. Too much building via excess protein, fat, starch and overeating tends to cause excess fat, weight (high cholesterol, fatty growths, tumors, etc.). Too much cleansing (salads, juices, cold drinks, etc.), tends to create excess water weight (edema, cellulite). Weak digestion is also a factor.

Digestion, acid, enzymes and bile, transforms food, nutrients into blood. Whatever food, fluids not digested, absorbed, become waste that is sent, moved down into the large intestine.

Too many cold, damp foods, drinks (soft dairy, salads, tropical fruits, juices, cold drinks, smoothies, shakes and sugar) dilute, weaken digestion, reducing nutrient absorption, blood, energy, heat, body temperature, while increasing waste (solid and liquid).

Strong digestion is the **ultimate fat burner** as it digests, burns excess protein, fat, cholesterol, sugar, water, etc.

Weak digestion burns, metabolizes **less fat**, cholesterol, etc. More tends to collect in the blood (clots, high cholesterol), arteries (plaque, atherosclerosis), arms, thighs (cellulite), etc.

Weak digestion burns, metabolizes **less water**. More water tends to collect in the stools (loose), ankles, arms (edema) and or reproductive organs (cysts, discharges, yeast infections, etc.).

Weak digestion burns, metabolizes **less sugar**. More tends to collect in the blood forcing the pancreas to overwork, and in the extreme, weaken. The pancreas regulates blood sugar and digestion, produces, secretes insulin, glucagon and digestive enzymes.

A weak, tired pancreas secretes (a) **less insulin, glucagon**, causing hypoglycemia (low blood sugar), hyperglycemia (high blood sugar), diabetes, and (b) **less digestive enzymes**, decreasing digestion, blood, nutrient absorption, while increasing waste.

The **hotter** middle diet is recommended for deficient, cold and damp conditions. Protein, fat especially animal, cooked vegetables, soups, stews, spices and exercise increases digestion, metabolism, burning of excess water weight. Decrease cold, damp foods (soft dairy), drinks and grains (processed). Be consistent with eating times. Dinner is the lightest, smallest meal. Large dinners and late night eating increase dampness, weight, constipation, insomnia, etc.

The **colder** middle diet, meal is recommended for, excess "fatty" high protein, high fat weight, growths, tumors, etc. Space or skip meals, especially dinner. Reduce animal protein, fat (red meat, veal, chicken) and processed grain (bread, noodles, cookies, chips, etc.). Processed **grains paste** the intestines in the same way cholesterol pastes the arteries. Vegetables (raw and cooked) and fruits cleanse excess protein, fat, paste, etc.

A wise man, woman controls the future. Control your refrigerator, kitchen cabinets by only stocking healthy foods (fruits, vegetables, yogurt, etc.). It is very hard to get fat on healthy foods, unlike junk foods, which are instantaneous weight. If you must eat junk, then go out and buy small amounts. Sometime you need a little junk to counter the junk of life. If you buy and stock large amounts of junk food, you will most likely eat large amounts and gain a lot of weight. You cannot eat what you do not stock.

Eat more during the day than at night. Digestion is naturally stronger during the day and weakest at night, which is why most cultures advise big (king) breakfast (protein, fat), big (prince) lunch and small (pauper) dinner. If you eat a big meal at night (after 6-7 P.M.), you will most likely wear it in the morning in your intestines, thighs, abdomen, arteries, etc.

Eat from hot (building) to cold (cleansing). Building (protein, fat), cooked foods, soups, spices, etc. stimulate digestion. Cleansing foods (salads, fruit) cool, moisten and clean (fiber) the intestines, help expel wastes, which is why they are generally eaten at the end.

If you crave sweets, snack on raw carrots, celery, oranges, apples and yogurt instead of pretzels, chips, cookies and ice cream. Eat until you are satisfied, full. Sweet is sweet. Which would you rather overeat? Make up your mind to lose weight, to eat less.

Think and write down all the stuff you do not like about being overweight, then read it every day. Resolve to be different, better, more disciplined, one meal, day at a time. Enjoy an empty stomach. You do not have to eat all the time, especially if you are not hungry.

Worms

Contaminated foods tend to cause worms. The hotter middle diet) less animal protein), bitter herbs (page 45), hot spices (cayenne) and seeds (pumpkin, sesame and sunflower) help counter worms. Medical consultation is also advised.

Yeast infection

The uterus and vagina are naturally moist. Too much moisture tends to create a clear or white vaginal discharge (leucorrhea), vaginitis and or yeast infection. Lower, colder body temperatures via long-term cold, damp diet (soft dairy, ice cream, juices, cold drinks, sugar, etc.) and chronic illness cool, moisten the uterus, vagina with excess mucous, yeast.

Normal body temperature (98.6°F) aided by the sun, protein, fat, digestion and exercise naturally heats and dries (regulates, thins bodily fluids) the body, uterus, vagina. Colder body temperatures thicken water. More info (Candidiasis pages 171- 173)

The hotter middle diet for cold, damp (cooked foods, spices, etc.) and raw cabbage juice is recommended.

Sage tea, vinegar douches, inserting a clove of garlic directly into the vagina or taking supplements containing caprylic acid can help cure today's yeast infections but not prevent their reoccurrence, which can only happen via change in diet. Bitter herbs (golden seal, mullein), in moderation may also be used, but are contraindicated when digestion and elimination are cold, damp. Check with your doctor first.

Yeast infection

- Stage 1: Dietary cause: long-term cold, damp diet: milk, yogurt, soft cheese, ice cream, salads, tropical fruits, juices, smoothies, shakes, sodas, cold drinks, sugar, desserts
- Stage 2: Digestion: abdominal bloating, gas
- Stage 3: Elimination: diarrhea, constipation
- Stage 4: Blood: fatigue, pain, pallor
- Stage 5: Circulation: coldness, mucous
- Stage 6: Organ: yeast infections, vaginitis

26

Case Histories

The following case histories were treated with the middle diet (pages 54- 58), adjusted accordingly.

1. **Anal Fissure** page 163

2. **Anemia** (blood deficiency): Several of my female customers, employees were suffering from blood deficiency, anemia (pale skin, diminished periods, thin hair and nails). All were vegetarians. It took me more than a year to convince them that their diets were anemic that they desperately needed to animal food. Once they started eating animal foods, they immediately felt better

3. **Anxiety** page 165

4. **Attention Deficit Disorder** (ADD) page 172

5. **Common cold** page 194

6. **Eczema** page 213

7. **GERD, GIRD** page 224

8. **Impotence** I had several male customer with sexual difficulties (inability to achieve or maintain an erection). Most were long-term (20+ years) coffee drinkers (3 cups+ per day). My advice was to give up coffee (caffeine drains the kidneys, jing). The few that gave up coffee saw their erections return. I also suffered from impotence. My condition however was caused by anemic diet, long-term vegetarian (15 years), not coffee. My erections came back once I started eating the hotter middle diet.

9. **Irritable Bowel Syndrome** (IBS) page 242

10. **Miscarriage** page 247

11. **Neuralgia** I met this young woman (professional ice skater); age 26 who came to my store, but could not stay; stand for too long because her feet would hurt. She had trouble walking and had to use a wheelchair on occasion. Her condition had started several years prior. She had seen many doctors, orthopedic surgeons, chiropractors, acupuncturists, blood work, x-rays, MRI, etc. No one was able to diagnose or help. She was blood deficient (long-term low protein, low fat and high carbohydrate diet). I recommended the hotter middle diet, red meat everyday, etc. A year later, she was able to walk, stand and skate without pain or fear.

12. **Post Nasal Drip** A friend had postnasal drip. Her diet was too cold (salads, fruits, cold drinks, etc.) causing excess water to accumulate and leak out her nose. I advised hotter middle diet. Her postnasal drip disappeared within days.

13. **Psoriasis** page 267

14. **Sinusitis** page 274

15. **Sore lower back** I occasionally develop lower and upper back pain whenever I eat or drink too many cold foods, drinks: ice cream, juices, etc. Every time I reduce or eliminate the source of coldness, in addition to increasing spicy foods, soups, the pain goes away.

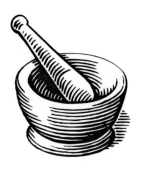

Section IV.
Daily Practices

27

Way of Breathing

The lungs control respiration exchange of gases, oxygen (O_2) and carbon dioxide (CO_2) between the body and the environment. The body is 65% oxygen, 18% carbon (C) 10% hydrogen (H) and 3% nitrogen (N). The brain consumes 20% of the body's oxygen (O) content.

Oxygen (pure chi) is the most important element, nutrient that one must continually breathe, in order to survive. Unconsciousness and death of brain, heart tissue, etc. occurs if the breath, breathing, blood, oxygen flow stops for more than a few minutes.

Carbon dioxide (gaseous waste) increases respiration, circulation, restlessness, etc. The art of breathing (and quality of air) is a vital part of exercise and meditation.

Photosynthesis ($6\ CO_2 + 6\ H_2O \rightarrow C_6H_{12}O_6 + 6\ O_2$) is the metabolic process whereby plants in the presence of sunlight, combine and transform carbon dioxide (exhaled by humans and animals) and water (H_2O) into carbohydrates ($C_6H_{12}O_6$): fruit, vegetables, grains, nuts, seeds and oxygen (O_2).

Air, oxygen produced by grass, plants, trees, is healthier, cleaner, more vibrant than air fouled, polluted by animals, humans, automobiles, industry, etc. Every home, if not located directly in nature should have plants. Plant produce exhale O_2 during the day and CO_2 at night and are usually kept out of the bedroom.

The lungs (hollow tubes, sacs) are naturally moist (includes mucous). Moisture, water facilitates the exchange of water-soluble gases: oxygen and carbon dioxide in the lungs, alveoli, blood (watery medium).

Colder body temperatures (less than 98.6°F) via long-term cold, damp diet or climate harden fluids in the lungs, throat, sinuses, etc. into excess mucous and phlegm, clogging, decreasing gas exchange while disrupting, shortening the breath.

Too little water via chronic blood deficiency (via long-term low protein, low fat and high carbohydrate diets), smoking or hot, dry climates weaken and dry the lungs, disrupt the breath.

There are two ways to breathe:

(1) Chest breathing (ribs expand and contract) is shallow, inefficient as it only uses the top third, half of the lungs shortening and speeding the breath to increase O_2 intake and CO_2 expulsion.

(2) Abdominal breathing (abdomen expands and contracts) is more efficient, using the entire capacity (top, middle and bottom) of the lungs, taking in more oxygen, and letting out more carbon dioxide (via the expansion and contraction of the abdomen), which in turn, requires less breaths (assuming the lungs are healthy, clear). Less breathing decreases heartbeat, relaxes the heart while calming the mind.

Deep abdominal breathing moves the diaphragm up and down, which massages the internal organs, increases digestion, absorption and elimination. The diaphragm is the partition of muscles and tendons that separate the chest cavity from the abdominal cavity.

Deep abdominal breathing is very simple. Inhalation: the breath is inhaled through the nose down into the lungs, bottom to top, via the expansion of the abdomen, front, sides and back. Holding the breath for ten to twenty seconds or more (comfortably, no strain) increases the absorption of oxygen. Holding the breath for long periods hurts the lungs.

Exhalation: the breath is exhaled out the mouth via contraction of the abdomen, which squeezes the lungs, bottom to top. A full exhalation complete with a "ha" sound helps empty the lungs of any stale air and is often practiced first thing in the morning to eliminate stagnant air in the lungs accumulated during the night when the body is less active.

Deep abdominal breathing decreases the amount of breaths per minute. There is a belief in Taoism that we are given a certain amount of breaths, just as if we are given a certain amount of jing. When those breaths expire, death ensues.

Most people inhale and exhale approximately ten times per minute. Slowing the breath to five to seven breaths per minute extends life. Respiration, like any function uses jing, blood; the more you breathe the more jing, blood you use, the faster you age. The less you breathe, the less jing, blood consumed, and the slower you age. Slowing the breath also calms the mind.

Fast, rapid, "bellow" breathing through the nose stimulates the heart, increasing circulation, energy, and body temperature, heat. Fast breathing also makes the mind and body restless, which is why slower breathing is used often as preparation for meditation, to help quiet, cool the mind.

Deep abdominal breathing can be done standing, sitting or lying down. Breathing exercise #1: Lay on your back, place your hands on your abdomen. Inhale into the lower abdomen, pushing it and the hands up, out. Exhale; use the hands to push in the abdomen. Practice for ten minutes.

Breathing exercise #2 Inhale slowly through nose to a count of ten, hold the breath to a count of ten and exhale via mouth to a count of ten. Repeat 20X four times a day, while sitting, walking, etc.

Deep abdominal breathing can also be done in reverse (embryonic). Embryonic breathing contracts the abdomen with the inhalation (front, side and back) and expands with the exhalation. This is the same way a baby, fetus breathes inside the womb, via the umbilicus. Many chi gung exercises use this style of breathing.

Deep abdominal breathing takes training. Do not practice deep abdominal breathing or hold the breath if you are a smoker, as you will damage your lungs, take pollutants deeper into the lungs. *Pregnant or menstruating women should not do deep abdominal breathing as it creates downward pressure on the fetus.*

Internal Exercise

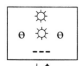

RIGHT SHOULDER	☼	**THYROID**
THYMUS	☼	HEART
RIGHT LUNG		LEFT LUNG
LIVER	☼	SPLEEN, **PANCREAS**
GALL BLADDER		STOMACH
RIGNT **ADRENAL**	☼	LEFT ADRENAL
RIGHT KIDNEY		LEFT KIDNEY
OVARIES, TESTES	☼	**SEX ORGANS**
LARGE INTESTINE		URINARY BLADDER

Everything is a reflection or energy. The body in traditional Chinese medicine (TCM) and Ayurveda is a reflection, interaction of the energies of heaven (stars, galaxies, etc.) and earth. The energy, force of heaven (Spirit, Intelligence) descends, enters the head at the **crown** and **medulla oblongata**, lowest part of brain stem and moves down the spine, where it interacts with the rising force of earth, which enters the body at the **perineum**: midway between the scrotum, vagina, and anus. These two forces **collide**, mix **seven** times producing seven spiritual energy centers, chakras (Sanskrit: wheels of energy) from which the glands, organs, meridians (energetic pathways), etc. develop. **Chi gung, yoga** and many martial arts consciously gather and direct energy up and down the spine and throughout the body via meridians, blood vessels, etc.

The seventh, crown chakra (thousand-pedaled lotus, throne of God) sits atop the skull produces the pineal gland (only found in humans), governs the spirit, universal consciousness.

The sixth chakra (third eye, Christ Consciousness) unique to human beings, is located in the frontal lobe between the eyes, eyebrows and connects to the medulla oblongata (mouth of God). It produces the pituitary gland, rules intellect and is the gateway to God. Brilliant light is seen when the third eye opens. "The light of the body is the eye: if therefore thine eye be single, thy whole body shall be full of light." Matthew 6:22.

The fifth, cervical chakra located at the base of the throat produces the thyroid gland, controls sound, speech, communication and the ability to be divinely calm. *Ether*

The fourth, dorsal chakra located in the middle of the chest produces the heart (circulation), lungs (respiration) and thymus gland and ability to love. "Blessed are the pure in heart for they shall see God" Mark 12:30 *Air*

The third, lumbar chakra located in the solar plexus produces the digestive organs (spleen, pancreas, stomach, liver, etc.). It controls energy and transformation. *Fire*

The second, sacral chakra located 3- 4 inches below navel produces the adrenal glands, kidneys and sexual organs. It controls reproduction, creativity and when conserved, harmonized, the ability to walk on water. *Water*

The first chakra is located in the coccyx. It produces and controls the excretory organs: urinary bladder and large intestine and is associated with the need to survive. Conserving and channeling moving energy in this chakra up the spine increases restraint as well as the ability to become intensely heavy, immovable. *Earth*

The meridians (energetic pathways, vessels connect the organs, spine, nerves, etc.) run up, down and around the body into the head, The **Du** and **Ren** Channels are the two major meridians. Both start in the **second chakra** and **transport jing.**

Ren Channel (Conception Vessel) is yin
- Originates in the lower abdomen (kidneys) and emerges at the **perineum** flowing up the front, midline of the body: abdomen, chest, throat and chin into the mouth (roof) where it ends.
- Stimulates, feeds the yin organs: liver, kidneys, spleen, heart, lungs and pericardium.

Du Channel (Governing Vessel) is yang
- Originates in the lower abdomen and emerges at the **perineum** flowing up the back, spine, back of the neck, head and forehead down the nose and into the mouth (roof) where is joins the Ren.
- Stimulates, feeds the yang organs: gall bladder, urinary bladder, stomach, small and large intestines and triple burner.

Placing the tongue against the roof of the mouth connects the Du and Ren. Every time you move, twist, bend, turn the head, neck, arms, legs, you also move, stimulate the meridians and related organs.

The arms, hands and fingers stimulate the **(1)** heart, **(2)** small intestine, **(3)** lungs, **(4)** large intestine, **(5)** pericardium (protective sac surrounding the heart) and **(6)** triple burner (TB): respiration, digestion and reproduction/ elimination.

The legs, feet and toes stimulate the **(7)** spleen, **(8)** stomach, **(9)** liver, **(10)** gall bladder (GB), **(11)** kidneys and **(12)** urinary bladder.

Exercise moves energy, blood, bones, muscles, organs, meridians, etc. **for better or worse.**

Fast moving exercises (sports) tend to deplete energy, misalign and or injure the bones, ligaments, etc. There are not many professional athletes beyond the age of 35, due to age, injuries. The young have greater flexibility, strength; healing ability and can generally easily suffer and repair physical abuse.

Slow moving and postural (sitting, standing) exercises (tai chi, yoga, chi gung, etc.) gently gather and direct energy often leaving one feeling refreshed, energized.

There are many stories of chi (energy) development, Eastern and Western. I once saw a Bill Moyer's special on television (PBS). It was about China, in particular, chi gung and martial arts. In one scene, there was an **eighty-year-old man (chi gung master) standing**, being pushed on the chest by a single line of twelve men (young, 20's), one behind another, pushing on the man in front. The old man did not budge, until ten minutes later when he appeared to dip, sink and suddenly straighten up, sending energy up and out his chest, at which time the twelve men explosively went flying backwards.

The Western story the scared young 100-pound mother is suddenly able to lift a two thousand pound car off her trapped child. The **power of chi** (cultivated via internal exercise) is greater than the muscles.

The **standing exercise** is the central, beginning and ending exercise of **chi gung** designed to conduct, gather and move heavens and earths force. The image of the standing exercise is the tree.

The **tree** is deeply rooted in the ground giving the upper, above ground tree its nutrition, strength and flexibility. It can be practiced outdoors or on a wooden floor for 20+ minutes, early in the morning and or late evening (negative ionic atmosphere). Clothing is loose; shoes are flat, comfortable and the stomach empty (two hrs after meal).

Chi Gung #1 Standing Exercise

1. The head is held as if suspended from a string attached to the crown. The eyes are opened slightly or closed fully. The tongue is held slightly against the roof of the mouth connecting the Du and Ren.

2. The chin tucked in, straightens the neck, vertebrae. There are 8 cervical nerves and 7 cervical vertebrae in the neck. Relax one vertebra at a time, from top to bottom

3. Shoulders pulled back, chest out, stomach in.

4. Spine: 12 thoracic nerves, vertebrae and 5 lumbar nerves, vertebrae. Relax one at a time, top to bottom.

5. Hips: 5 sacral nerves and vertebra. Tilt the hips in to straighten and relax the lower spine

6. The knees are bent and extend directly over, but not beyond the toes (may cause injury). The legs are shoulder's width apart, and the feet parallel or slightly pointed outwards. The weight of the body is evenly distributed left and right, front and back

7. The arms, hands hang loose, near, touching the outside if the thighs, or held in front (1) parallel with the chest (upper burner, circulation, respiration), (2) below the ribs (middle burner, digestion) or (3) below the navel (lower burner, reproduction, elimination) as if holding a large beach ball. Fingers, tips point to each other and barely touch.

8. Close the eyes and imagine, feel heaven's force, energy sinking unimpeded down through the head, brain, spine, back of the legs and feet into the ground. Then feel earth's energy rise up the feet, spine into the brain. Opening the Energy Gates by B. K. Frantzis gives a complete, detailed explanation and exercise program. The standing exercise, while complete, does not, stretch, bend the body, bones, meridians, which is why additional exercises are performed

Chi Gung #2 Look Left, Look Right

1. Stand in a horse stance (standing exercise, 1- 6 with the feet spread greater than shoulder's width). The arms relaxed, held at the sides. The eyes look straight ahead.

2. Inhale deeply into the lower abdomen, then exhale and slowly turn the head (chin parallel to the shoulders) to the left. Look, stare over the left shoulder. Inhale and return to the center. Exhale and turn the head slowly to the right. Stare over the right shoulder (benefits the eyes, liver). Inhale and return to the center. This is one complete rotation. Repeat 6- 12 times.

3. You can also bend the head forward, down (exhale) and backwards, up (inhale). This increases the circulation of blood and chi between the head, neck and rest of the body. It mimics the head movements of the turtle (symbol of longevity), which can live 100 years +.

Chi Gung #3 Adjusting Triple Burner

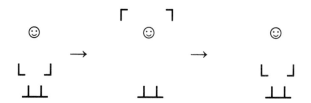

1. Assume the horse stance and bring the hands close to each other, palms facing up three inches below the navel. The hands, fingers can be interlaced or separate.

2. Inhale deeply into the abdomen and slowly raise the arms, hands out in front of the body in an arc that passes over the head. The eyes stare straight ahead but follow the hands, palms, which eventually rotate, face away and point upwards. Hold for a few seconds.

3. Exhale and slowly lower the arms, hands, rotating the palms down (eyes following, until level), back to their original position. Repeat 6- 12 times.

4. Variation: Coordinate, lift your heels off the floor as you push your palms up, and then lower the heels to the ground, as the palms, arms lower. This exercise moves chi from the lower burner (kidneys, sex organs, large intestine) to the middle (spleen, stomach, liver, etc.) to the upper (lungs, heart). The three burners, energy centers transform chi, blood and waste.

Chi Gung #4 Uniting Fire and Water

Step One. Raise the chi   Step Two. Lower the chi

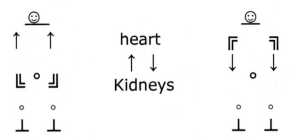

1. Stand in a horse stance. Bring the hands 3" below the navel*, close together, fingertips pointing towards one another, palms facing up. The eyes look straight ahead. Inhale deep into the abdomen and raise the palms, breath up to the solar plexus (below the sternum). Hold the breath and let the chi gather. Turn the palms over, exhale and push the chi back down to the lower abdomen*. Repeat 6- 12 times.

This exercise unites, moves energy up and down the spine, between the heart (fire) and the kidneys (water). It also helps relieve, move abdominal and intestinal pain, clogging.

Chi Gung #5 Adjust Stomach and Spleen

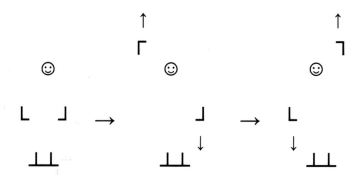

1. Stand in a horse stance with the hands, 3" below the navel, palms face up held close together, fingertips almost touching

2. Inhale deeply in the lower abdomen Raise the right hand, palm in an arc away from the body as it rises overhead. The palm rotates, pushes up as it rises so that it faces up when fully extended.

3. The left palm (stationary) also rotates so that it is facing, pushing down. The right hand pushes up, the left hand down. Hold this position for a few seconds. The pushing of the hands arches stretches the chest and abdomen. Exhale and return both hands to their original position.

4. Inhale and raise, push the left hand, palm, overhead, facing up, while rotating, pushing the right hand, palm downward. The left hand pushes up and the right hand down. Exhale and return to the starting position. This is one complete rotation. Repeat 6- 12X.

This exercise stimulates the spleen and stomach (meridians pass through the abdomen), helps relieve upset stomach, abdominal bloating, overeating, anal pain and constipation (moves the bowels down).

Chi gung #6 Bend forward, Bend Backward

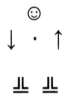

1. Stand in a horse stance. The arms are relaxed along the sides of the body, legs, knees slightly bent. Breathe deeply, quietly for 1 minute. Exhale and slowly bend over. Keep the back straight and the head slightly raised as you bend over, one vertebra at a time. The lower back bends first, then middle and upper.

2. Relax in this position. If possible, try to grab beneath the toes, between the balls of the feet or around the ankles and pull the head, body towards the legs. Kidney energy enters the body between the balls of the feet (acupuncture point: bubbling wells). Grabbing this point stimulates the kidneys.

3. Inhale and raise up, vertebra by vertebra from bottom to top of the spine until you are upright. Then place the hands on the lower back (for support), exhale and lean backwards. Inhale and return to the starting position. Repeat 6- 12 times.

This exercise is beneficial to the kidneys, lower back, abdomen and spine. The body, small of the back (where the kidneys are located) opens up when the body bends over, which relaxes the kidneys.

Chi gung #7 Turning the Waist

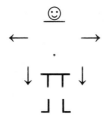

1. Assume the horse stance (knees bent; hips and chin tucked in, feet parallel or turned slightly out. The arms hang loosely at the sides or with hands on the hips. The eyes look straight ahead. The hips, knees and legs face forward but do not turn, twist. In this exercise, the upper body twists, turns the waist not the hips.

2. Inhale deeply into the lower abdomen, exhale and turn the upper body slowly to the right. The head does not turn. Eyes look straight ahead. Hold for a few seconds. Inhale and return to the center. Repeat to the left side. This is one complete rotation. Repeat 6- 12 times. Turning the waist stimulates, opens the kidneys.

Chi gung #8 Lifting the Heals

1. Stand in a horse stance with the arms at the sides of the body. Breathe deeply and quietly. Inhale and raise the heals off the ground, standing on the balls of the feet. Hold for a few seconds. Exhale and slowly lower the heals back to the ground. Repeat 6- 10 times. This exercise stimulates the kidneys (Bubbling wells).

The last, final exercise is always the standing exercise. The arms, hands are held out in front of the lower abdomen in order to direct, gather chi back into the lower abdomen, kidneys, jing. Stand for 5- 10 minutes +/-.

Do not do chi gung in the wind, when windy (wind scatter). Chi gung can be done by young or old. Please seek out a teacher, book or video, as this chapter is only an introduction. Success comes with training and discipline (practice, practice). Please consult your doctor before attempting any new exercise program

Resources
- *Five Animal Chi Gung* by Ken Cohen (video)
- *Taoist Eight Treasures* by Maoshing Ni (video)
- *Eight Pieces of Brocade* by Dr. Yang Jwing Ming
- *Beginning Chi Gung* by S. Kuei and S. Comee
- *Opening the Energy* Gates by B. K. Frantzis

Appendix

Bibliography

1. Anderson, Bob, **Stretching**, Shelter Publications, Inc. 1980
2. Beinfield, Harriet, L. Ac, Effrem Korngold, L. Ac. O.M.D., **Between Heaven and Earth, A Guide To Chinese Medicine**, Ballantine Books, 1991
3. Bensky, Dan and Andrew Gamble, **Chinese Herbal Medicine, Materia Medica**, Eastland Press, 1986
4. Chang, Dr. Steven T., **The Great Tao**, Tao Publishing, 1985
5. **The Tao of Balanced Diet**, 1986
6. **The Complete System of Self-Healing, Internal Exercises**
7. Cohen, Ken, **The Way of Qigong,** Ballantine Books, 1997
8. Flaws, Bob, **Prince Wen Hui's Cook, Chinese Dietary Therapy**, Paradigm Publications, 1983
9. **The Tao of Healthy Eating,** Blue Poppy Press, 1998
10. Frantzis, B.K., **Opening the Energy Gates of Your Body**, First Atlantic N. Publishing Co., 1993
11. Foreign Language Press, **Chinese Acupuncture and Moxibustion**, Beijing, 1987
12. Heinerman, John, **Encyclopedia of Nuts, Berries and Seeds**, Parker Publishing Co., 1995
13. **Encyclopedia of Fruits, Vegetables and Herbs**,
14. **The Complete Book of Spices**, Keats Publishing Inc. 1983
15. Holmes, Peter, **The Energetics of Western Herbs, Integrating Western and Oriental Herbal Medicine Traditions**, Artemis, 1989
16. Kuei, Steven and Stephen Comee, **Beginning Qigong,** Charles E. Tuttle Publishing Co. Inc., 1993
17. Lam Kam Chuen, **The Way of Energy**, Gaia Books Limited, 1991

18. Lu, Henry C., **Chinese System of Food Cures**, Sterling Publishing Co. Inc. 1986
19. **Chinese Foods for Longevity, The Art of Long Life**, 1990
20. Maciocia, Giovanni, **The Foundations of Chinese Medicine,** Churchill Livingston, 1989
21. Masahiro, Oki, **Zen Yoga Therapy,** Japan Publications Inc., 1979
22. Rothenberg, Dr. Mikel A., M.D. and Chapman, Charles F., **Dictionary of Medical Terms,** Barron's Educational Series, Inc. 2000
23. Tierra, Michael, **Planetary Herbology**, Lotus Press, 1988
24. Dr. Yang Jwing- Ming, **The Eight Pieces of Brocade,** Yang's Martial Arts Association, 1988
25. Yeung, Him-Che, L. Ac., **Handbook of Chinese Herbs and Formulas, Volume 1**, Institute of Chinese Medicine, 1983

About the Author

Richard G. Heft was born in NYC, NY (1952). He attended the University of Pittsburgh (1971-1974) and graduated with a B.A. in political science. In 1984, he purchased a small health food store in Hollywood, FL, renaming it Food and Thought (1984-2001); attended, graduated the Acupressure Acupuncture Institute, Miami, FL (1989-91), with a degree in acupuncture, nutrition, and massage, licensed professionally, Acupuncture Physician (FL 1992-2002). For ten years or more, questioned and counseled his customers (400+ per week), always asking the same question, "What do you eat for breakfast, lunch and dinner?" Wrote and published **Hot and Cold Health** (c) 2003, **Hot and Cold Diseases** (c) 2008, combing both into **Hot and Cold Health and Disease** (c) 2009; Personal hobbies: meditation, chi gung, reading, walking, spending time outdoors, talking to my neighbors, etc.

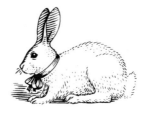

CPSIA information can be obtained at www.ICGtesting.com
Printed in the USA
BVOW08s1609091013

333325BV00002B/216/P